PREVENTION MYTHS

Why Stress Tests Can't Predict Your Heart
Attack and Which Tests Actually Do

Ford Brewer, MD, MPH

Todd C Eldredge PHD, MPH, MBA

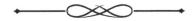

PREVENTION MYTHS

Why Stress Tests Can't Predict Your Heart Attack and Which Tests Actually Do

ABSTRACT

Nearly nine million times each year, patients are submitted to excessive radiation and invasive procedures to see if they are at risk for a heart attack or stroke. Unfortunately, these tests only catch those whose condition is bad enough to warrant an invasive procedure.

The probability of false negative and false positive results is just way too high. They do absolutely nothing for the vast majority whose conditions can only be treated with effective medical care.

The few tests that catch >98% of the heart attacks and strokes before they occur have not been recommended to them by their physician for consideration. This book addresses that concern and tells you which tests could help you to prevent that heart attack or stroke, in time to treat them medically and not surgically.

Ford Brewer, MD, MPH
Todd C Eldredge PHD, MPH, MBA
fbrewer@prevmedheartrisk.com
todd@cardiorisk.com

Healthy Heart Publishing
9677 South 700 East, Sandy UT. 84020
www.healthyheartco.com
www.prevmedheartrisk.com
vs 1.6

Cover design: Evolve Global Publishing
Library of Congress Cataloging-in-Publication Data
Brewer, Ford; Eldredge, Todd
PREVENTION MYTHS: Why Stress Tests Can't Predict Your Heart Attack and Which Tests Actually Do
Ford Brewer, MD, MPH and Todd C. Eldredge, PHD, MPH, MBA
Pages cm
Interior v7 / Font name - Minion Pro

ASIN: B096XD1ZRD (Amazon Kindle)
ISBN: 979-8-51826-263-8 (Amazon Print)
ISBN: 978-1-63944-113-6 (Ebook)
ISBN: 978-1-63848-013-6 (IngramSpark Paperback)
ISBN: 978-1-63848-014-3 (IngramSpark Hardcover)
ISBN: 978-1-63944-113-6 (Smashwords)

1. Medical books – Diseases - Cardiovascular.
2. Health, Fitness & Dieting – Diseases & Physical Ailments - Heart Disease
3. Medical Books – Administration & Policy - Health Risk Assessment
4. Medical Books - Internal Medicine - Cardiology

Printed in the United States of America

Table of Contents

This book is dedicated to Tim Russert and all those other human beings that relied too much on stress tests. Hopefully, this book and the new research on which it is based, will help steer us back to good health.

For Heidi, Janice, and our families

You ALL are our happiest thoughts – may you always have good health!

Prevention Myths

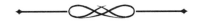

ABOUT THE AUTHORS

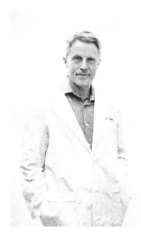

Ford **Brewer, MD, MPH:** Ford is the author of over two dozen peer-reviewed medical science articles. He also runs a YouTube channel on Preventive Medicine with over 90,000 subscribers. He started his career as a physician in the Emergency Department over 30 years ago. It quickly became clear that the injuries and diseases that brought people into his emergency departments should have been prevented. So, he went back for more training, this time in Preventive Medicine. He did well and ended up running the post-graduate program at Johns Hopkins.

Since then, he has been a career medical director, supervising medical staff programs. Several of these had over 1,000 physicians. Dr. Brewer now runs a program (PrevMed) which educates and treats hundreds of patients, savings lives by preventing heart attacks, strokes, and blindness. Each week there are commenters on the YouTube channel expressing gratitude for saving their own lives through critical prevention techniques. By far the most common comments provide documentation of previously unrecognized diabetes or prediabetes.

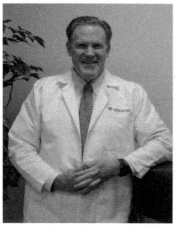

Todd Eldredge, MBA, MPH, PhD: Eldredge is the author of the #1 International Best-Selling book "Cardiovascular Wellness Management Success Plan" and an active researcher, involved in many CIMT-related research projects. Todd spent many years developing performance-based testing protocols to demonstrate operator-dependent coefficients of variability and testing reproducibility. He spent 10 years at what is now Sanofi-Pasteur where he ran a Pediatric Vaccine Business Unit. Eldredge has a BSBA, MBA, and MPH degrees and a PhD in cardiovascular-epidemiology.

Eldredge is the Founder and CEO of CardioRisk Laboratories, an international heart attack, and stroke prevention company. Eldredge also co-founded the WellnessVIP (Vascular Improvement Program) (WellnessVIP, Inc.; www.wellnessvip.org) which integrates phenotypical, genotypical, and physical diagnostic testing to diagnose at-risk patients, optimize their care, and monitor the efficacy of treatment in patients with increased cardiovascular risk.

Prior to CardioRisk and WellnessVIP, Eldredge was a founder and/or senior executive of several bio and technical companies with roots in quality, technology, and biologicals whose combined success exceeded $100MM in annual revenues.

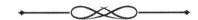

WHY WE WROTE THIS BOOK:

- FORD

Blind Alleys - "Listen to the patient. He's telling you the diagnosis," versus "Test, don't guess."

These two quotes have been big issues for me throughout my career. The debate surrounds testing. In my training and later, as an emergency physician, I developed a strong opinion that doctors did not listen well to patients. They relied on X-rays, labs and other tests. That surprised me. I had expected to find a lot of curious people when I went to medical school. Instead, it seemed that medical school, during my time, attracted a lot of people that were better at memorizing and test-taking than thinking or listening. The problem is not that medicine is boring. Medical diagnostic mysteries can be fascinating. The television series whodunit HOUSE was the most watched TV show in 2008. It was the personality type that got into medical school during my era. I kept thinking that if doctors would just listen more to their patients - and test less - they would get the right diagnosis. Long after I left Hopkins, I found a friend in a quote attributed to William Osler.

"JUST LISTEN TO THE PATIENT. HE'S TELLING YOU THE DIAGNOSIS."

The story goes like this. Osler was running grand rounds as he often did in the amphitheater at Hopkins. A student physician was taking a history. He was not doing very well, at least according to Osler, who interrupted the young doctor. "Just listen to the patient. He's telling you the diagnosis."

BLIND ALLEYS - FALSE POSITIVE RESULTS ON TESTS THAT NEVER SHOULD HAVE BEEN ORDERED

American medicine is choked with examples of unnecessary medical care. We will cover overuse in detail later in this book. A simple study of lab tests indicated, that 85% were unnecessary, squandering $86 million in one study alone (Allen 2018). Those studies always frustrated me. They seemed to miss the bigger picture that the waste was often not the study itself, but the blind alleys and pain caused by false positive studies that never should have been ordered in the first place. We will talk later about false positive stress tests leading to cardiac catheter procedures.

"TEST, DON'T GUESS"

So, you can imagine my reaction when I first heard the battle cry of the Bale Doneen CV prevention community, "Test, Don't Guess". To me, it sounded like the worst of medicine; too much money, wasted technology; and doctors that believed everything a test result said. But I suspended my disbelief to try the experience . . . and I learned something. I could not deny the results they were getting.

The patients were reversing their cardiac risks. I was seeing much higher rates of significant lifestyle changes. By significant, I'm referring to changes comparable to 20-pound weight loss or more. It is clear that much of this is a thing called selection bias. Selection bias is correlation between the selection criteria and the outcome. For example, I am not saying that the increase success rate is entirely due to increased testing. It is clear that paying $4,000 for a Bale Doneen evaluation selects for individuals already motivated to make big lifestyle changes. It is impossible to say how much of this is selection bias and how much of it is the testing.

SHOW, DON'T TELL

Janice is taking a writing class for authors. Her first few classes seemed to be on the same subject. They keep telling her that good authors "show, they don't tell." If you want someone to believe something, you don't tell them. You show them. That is the value of lab tests. As a patient, you are no longer hearing some expert telling you an opinion. You are seeing exactly what is actually happening in your body.

- TODD

Although I have shared this story previously and in many different formats and on many different stages – it is still relevant. Great musicians often include repeat covers of their songs on subsequent albums – so please forgive me for retelling this story. It is an important part of who I am and why I do what I do and there are only so many ways to tell this story.

While in my freshman year of high school, my mind was occupied by many of the activities and curriculum that consume the thoughts of a typical 15-year-old young man. Sports; friends; scholarship… well, … not so much; girls… (definitely!); the movie coming out next month; music on the radio and more specifically, who would win Casey Kasem's top 40 this weekend; these were the types of ideas that occupied my mind as best as I can recall in the winter of 1977.

My mom and dad had six children. My younger brother Stephen died at birth leaving my parents with five otherwise healthy children. My older brother David and I had what I consider to be a typical sibling relationship. We quarreled, we fought, we even knocked each other out at one point, but within the confines of what I consider a typical sibling relationship was a deep and abiding love and friendship for each other that only two brothers separated by a few years of age can know or understand.

My parents owned a baby blue 1970 Chevy Kingswood Wagon - a station wagon with that famous Chevy 350 V-8 engine. It drank gas… at about 6 MPG by the time I was driving it. This car had been relegated and assigned to the unfortunate position of being the primary family learning fleet vehicle, as it was the car designated for use by each of my siblings when we learned to drive. I say designated because it never really made it past my own experience… and I was #2 in the family birth order.

As the first sibling to reach the age of 16, David got to drive it first. He managed to put several dents in the car in the form of minor fender-benders, causing great consternation to those of us who had yet to matriculate through a proper driver's education course, nor even reach a legal age in order to take it for a test drive.

One of the biggest arguments I had with my brother concerned his negligent driving habits and the affect those habits may have had on my future opportunity to drive, let alone my potential access to a functioning vehicle.

Having established that I was not yet old enough to drive legally, my primary mode of transportation was the city bus. My daily weekday routine consisted of arriving at the appropriate bus stop just in time, but not a minute too soon, to catch the scheduled route and arrive at my appointed destination in time to converse with friends who found themselves in a similar situation.

Daily I dreamed and counted the days until I could at least share the family's vehicle with my brother, or even better, until the day he left for college and I could inherit the asset entirely for my own enjoyment. Such was my station in life in February of 1977.

Upon arriving home on a Thursday afternoon of that year, I began my near religious weekday ritual of watching my favorite cartoons and sitcoms: Gilligan's Island, Batman, and the Flintstones were a few of my favorites. It is a bit sequacious to remind some that there were no internet, iTunes, Netflix, and only a few channels of cable television were available in 1977 - and we didn't have that luxury.

Somewhere during this standardized routine, a call came through the family phone (we also didn't have cell or wireless phones in those days - they were all corded and rotary dial.) My mother answered and upon completion she casually explained that David had been in an accident and she had to go get him.

"Great", I remember thinking . . . "He's wrecked the car again." After all, we had been through this routine before . . . several times. I didn't give it too much more thought that that. However, as the sitcoms and cartoons continued long past my standard routine, and into the early evening, I became acutely aware of a nervous and foreboding feeling that had slowly crept into my conscience. By 6:00 PM it had fully taken center stage.

At length I realized that my parents had simply been gone for too long. As the minutes turned into hours, that sense of fear and foreboding increased, and genuine worry began to fill my mind as I openly acknowledged the concern I was trying desperately to ignore. What could possibly be taking my parents so long?

Eventually I heard the family car pulling up to the curb and the unmistakable sound of the car doors opening and closing. However, these somewhat routine sounds were accompanied by what, at first blush, sounded like a maniacal and hideous laugh. I subsequently, but quickly recognized it as the sound of my mother crying hysterically. "Trouble . . . big trouble" I thought.

I sprinted down the stairs of our home and out the front door, off the porch and down the cement stairs that led to the porch where I met my parents. My Dad was practically carrying my Mother. I will never forget the painful expressions emoting from their long faces. As we met physically on the sidewalk my father managed to emit a broken whisper of despair and he said to me: "Son, . . . David is dead, . . . he was killed in a car accident."

Unless you have personally experienced something like this - there is no way to describe the weight of the impact of those words. A kick in the gut doesn't begin to properly describe the sensation - though they would be in the correct quadrant of pain. The words alone literally knocked me off my feet and I fell to my knees in shock and despair as my mind grasped for meaning and I tried to wrap my young mind around what it meant. Truthfully, it would take years to process.

There simply are no words to describe the sudden and tragic loss of life of a family member. Though millions have gone through similar events, and many millions more will undoubtedly experience similar emotions . . . my experience was unique to me . . . as I am sure their experiences are completely, and unequivocally unique to them.

There was nothing I, nor anyone else, could have done to prevent this tragedy. My brother was a passenger in a car driven by someone else, along with five of his friends. The truck that ran into them, full of salty sand to spread on the slippery streets of our snow-covered city, was also driven by a well-intentioned driver.

I suppose it is a natural element of any disaster to attempt to assign blame. I mean, how could this possibly happen? What could have been done differently? At the end of the day, there are no real answers to those questions . . . and even if there were, I am not sure it would bring any comfort to those who mourn the loss of a loved one.

For me - this experience is one of several which shape and inform many of the thoughts, feelings, and motivations I have relating to the sanctity and value of life, the importance of telling people we love them, and of sharing what they mean to us, and how paramount it is to treasure time with loved one . . . because we simply never know when the fragility of life will tip the scales and those we care deeply about will disappear from this realm we can see and touch.

Now please don't think after reading this that I am a mere sentimentalist. I am also a realist who embraces science and scientific method. I have read the book of life, and I understand that it is a tragic love story. I mean . . . we all know how it ends. Spoiler alert: none of us are getting out of this thing called life alive.

Having said that, I also believe that it is noble and meritorious to engage in those activities that extend the quality and quantity of life. Even though the ending is inevitable . . . the importance of being able to write a better, more prolonged, happier ending cannot be understated. As one of my physician friends named Gerry put it, "We are engaged in the art of adding play time minutes to the game of life." I love that!

In the case of my older brother, there was literally nothing that I could have done that would have altered his ending. This is tragic - but I can accept it as a metaphysical certainty.

By now I can imagine you must be thinking, "Yes, but what does this have to do with the price of beans in China???" . . . or more specifically, "What does it have to do with heart attack and stroke prevention?"

Let us fast forward a few decades to bring this discussion full circle. Contextual meaning is relevant to understanding where people are coming from. This backdrop should shed additional light on why all this matters, or at least why it matters to me.

As a function of my education and professional associations I became acquainted with technology that showed promise in its ability to identify those at increased risk for heart attack and stroke in time to treat and prevent the disease medically and not surgically. I was aware that many people (86% of those who have a heart attack or stroke) never make it or get the opportunity to qualify for a surgical intervention because the first sign or symptom they had was a massive heart attack or stroke. Over half of those, whose first symptom or sign was the heart attack, die from the event. Waiting for signs, symptoms, or enough arterial obstruction for the cardiologist to intervene is just not a rational option. If we want to put a dent in the current morbidity and mortality statistics, then we MUST do a better job of identifying people at risk, and we need them to take aggressive action. The earlier we can act, the more likely we can preserve human life.

I was enthralled with this technology from the very first minute I was exposed to it. I was surprised at the vast amount of research that had already been published by the time I was introduced. I could not contain my enthusiasm to better understand this technology.

Eventually I was able to receive one-on-one training from one of the men who pioneered the method, Dr. Gene Bond. Dr. Bond is one of the most knowledgeable people I ever met on any subject. He is especially gifted with regards to his knowledge about atherosclerosis and other arterial diseases, the tools used to image and assess the disease, its etiology and pathophysiological pathways. Dr. Bond's curriculum vitae is a book in and of itself. It took me nearly five years of concerted effort just to read through and absorb the volumes of his published research.

Dr. Bond was a co-author of the ARIC (the Atherosclerosis Risk In Communities - Chambless 97) and many other landmark studies. He had been a professor of medicine at Wake Forest school of medicine for nearly 30 years. He was a gifted pathologist with a masters in anatomy. It was a highlight of my life to have been mentored by him and to have spent nearly 10 years learning from his experience.

To be truthful, it is unlikely I will ever know everything Dr. Bond knew about this disease - but one hopes that one has at least understood the most crucial and important details uncovered during the time I was fortunate enough to have spent by his side. Beyond that, and somewhat parenthetically, Dr. Bond is a compassionate, kind, and caring human being who was a gentleman in every human interaction I ever witnessed.

Sometime during my training, and after having demonstrated proficiency in the method via a double-blind, performance-based certification, I took an ultrasound machine with me to my parents' home for a Thanksgiving holiday. I was anxious to share some of my knowledge about this technology, and I was anxious to demonstrate for my siblings that they were all healthy. I expected nothing less. My family supported my enthusiasm. Each member agreed to let me examine their carotid arteries.

My next younger brother is seven years younger than me. He is a commercial airline pilot. In my mind, he was the picture of health. At the time of my first scan of his arteries, he was in his 30's, he was running five miles daily, five times weekly. He had minimal body fat. He was tall and slender and seemed to have a relatively stress-free life (easy for me to say).

Prevention Myths

Upon beginning an ultrasonic mapping process of his arteries my eyes caught a glimpse of something. Closer examination confirmed he had a large, soft plaque in his right carotid artery. I instantly understood the ramifications of this finding.

Research has shown that 84% of the lesions this size were likely to rupture within 10 years (Belcarro 2001). Further research has shown that the soft core was many times more likely to rupture than a hard plaque (Honda 2004).

I remembered feeling that same sense of foreboding and dread I had experienced when waiting to hear about my older brother's condition. I simply could not bear the thought of prematurely losing another brother - especially to a disease that was nearly 100% preventable. Not on MY WATCH! To make a long story short - I was able to get my brother connected with an expert in treating this disease and preventing potential events.

It has now been nearly two decades since I first found this lesion in my brother's carotid artery. He still flies commercially. He has raised his two children to adulthood. He has weathered the stressful storms I have learned are inherent to commercial aviation (buyouts, furloughs, working abroad) and has managed to stay healthy and free from even the slightest sign of cardiovascular disease. He has managed his prediabetes and is likely to live a long and prosperous life. It is highly unlikely he will die from CV disease.

To me this last story underscores the reality of the disease - it is not just a case study for those who are touched by its reach. To those affected by its insidious tentacles, the disease is real. This disease impacts real people, real jobs, real families, and real incomes. It is not merely a case study to be listened to in an auditorium of doctors. I cannot detach myself from the familial aspects and its heightened potential for emotional impact.

I was unable to do anything about my older brother's death, but I have been able to do something about the lives of friends, family members, and associates to help extend the length and quality of their lives. What happened to my two brothers motivates me every day. These events keep reminding me that disease prevention matters. Cardiovascular disease has impacted my parents, my siblings, my aunts, uncles, cousins, friends and family. It has also touched me in a personal way. My own arteries needed aggressive therapy.

This disease is rampant. Everyone I contact knows someone who keeled over unexpectedly from a heart attack. Most of these deaths were preventable. Until the medical community gets more effective at identifying risk, further progress will be hindered. It is my greatest desire to keep our medical and research communities focused on mitigating death and long-lasting sequelae relating to this pernicious disease. I believe it is worthy of my life's effort and so it remains the focus of my time and energy.

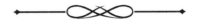

INTRODUCTION

A TYPICAL STANDARD OF CARE TESTING TRAGEDY

April 29th, 2008, was a beautiful day in Washington, DC. It was four weeks after the Cherry Blossom Festival. The weather outside was mostly sunny, with occasional clouds. The temperature was in the 50s most of the day, with a high of 62.

Michael Newman is a well-known internist, a doctor to Washington's elite. One of those elite patients—a top figure in his field—was on the treadmill for a stress test.

Dr. Newman had suggested that the patient lose weight. But doctors always do that. Yes, this patient was getting older—now 58. Middle-aged men often gain weight. But this had not negatively impacted this patient's work. His job required lunch and dinner meetings with national and even world leaders. He had to be focused, not distracted with dieting.

He was not ignoring Dr. Newman's advice. He was trying to lose weight, but it was difficult. He knew what he had to do. He told the doc he was going to do it when the right time came, and he meant it.

He and his doc both knew he had coronary artery disease. The patient had a positive Coronary Calcium Score years ago. There was no chest pain. Dr. Newman correctly pointed out that the best way to handle coronary artery disease was not with stents but with lifestyle and medications. The doctor adjusted this patient's blood pressure medication.

Other risk factors which were assessed were favorable for this patient. His family history was not ominous. He did not smoke. Even though they had adjusted his medications, his blood pressure was under control. Total cholesterol and LDL values were not demonstrably high.

Dr. Newman also used the Framingham standards to estimate the CV risk of this patient. The patient's Framingham risk score was less than 10% for an event over the next ten years. For a 58-year-old patient with coronary artery disease, high blood pressure, and a weight problem, the prognosis was not too bad. A stress test that day incorrectly confirmed a good prognosis. These two preventative risk assessments, on this patient, demonstrate the often-fatal flaws of these tools.

Passing the stress test was a relief. The patient did not believe he had a problem that needed immediate, drastic or surgical attention. As he had told his physician many times, he did plan to deal with his weight "when the time is right." The patient returned to his life and work, putting off the weight loss. When his son Luke graduated from college, the family visited Italy to celebrate. He returned to Washington DC on Friday the 13th to prepare for the weekly edition of his nationally syndicated show which would air on Sunday, June 15th. This was six weeks following his negative stress test.

While recording voice-overs in the studio that day, he collapsed and died. We provide, below, the transcript from the NBC News Special Report of the incident.

TRANSCRIPT OF NBC NEWS SPECIAL REPORT, JUNE 13TH, 2008:

Andrea Mitchell - "Joining me now is a very close, close friend (pause) - a close friend of Tim Russert's, who was with him, and - Dr. Newman, you & I, we know each other, (pause) and both know Tim, but you had the sad duty of being with him today in the ER. I don't know what you can share."

Dr. Michael Newman - (exhales, then speaks). "It's a, uh (a long pause),

Andrea Mitchell - Talk a bit about Tim, and talk a bit about cardiac disease, and sudden cardiac arrest.

Dr. Michael Newman - Tim had coronary artery disease. He had no symptoms but asymptomatic coronary disease, as we see in many men and women. His risk factors were well-managed. He was well-informed. He did his best with respect to diet, exercise, lifestyle. His blood pressure was well-controlled. His cholesterol fractions were optimal. He had a stress test on April 29th, got to a very high level of exercise. He was quite pleased with his performance as we were.

This morning, like most mornings, he got on his treadmill and was always excited about how he pushed himself. Uh, these events, these sudden cardiac events, occur without warning. There is no way to anticipate or detect them. An hour before this happened, he could have had a stress test, and it would have been perfectly normal. The reason why these events occur is because you have rupture of cholesterol plaque in the wall of the coronary artery. And that causes a sudden cardiac, coronary thrombosis, which results in a heart attack, and the injury causes a fatal - in this instance - ventricular arrhythmia."

Andrea Mitchell - "And this was a blood clot when you say in the coronary..."

Dr. Newman - "A concern that we had was that perhaps this was related to a pulmonary embolus, because Tim had flown on Sunday to Rome for Luke's birthday and graduation and turned around. We did the autopsy to determine the cause of death. An autopsy is important despite all the technology and scans and imaging that we have. The autopsy showed that Tim had an enlarged heart and significant coronary artery disease in the left anterior descending coronary artery. And we could actually see a fresh clot right in the coronary artery. That was the coronary thrombosis that triggered the coronary event and the arrhythmia from which he died."

Andrea Mitchell - "Dr. Newman, help us with this because we know him as such a vigorous, active man. He'd just flown back. He'd just taped a broadcast this morning, and was downstairs here, recording the opening sequence for MEET THE PRESS, and collapsed. Was there anything - the EMT guys got here very quickly. Is there anything they could have done? They worked on him for 10 minutes."

Dr. Newman - "The, uh, as soon as we got the - a few moments, it was recognized that Tim was in trouble. And one of the interns here, who's certified in CPR, along with some of the staff here, began CPR. And that was helpful. And a defibrillator is what makes the difference. In this sudden cardiac arrest, the use of a defibrillator - which they were in the process of doing - is important. The

Prevention Myths

DC EMS arrived promptly, and they immediately defibrillated Tim. And they actually did it three times in transporting him to Sibley hospital."

Andrea Mitchell - "Is there, in the brief time that we have left. Let me just clarify. This was a known condition?"

Dr. Newman - "He was known to have coronary artery disease. There are many men and women that have coronary artery disease. It was well-managed. There was a recent study, the COURAGE Trial, that showed that medical management of coronary artery disease is the way to go."

Andrea Mitchell - "And, by the time he got, he was never resuscitated?"

Dr. Newman - "He was never resuscitated. The defibrillation efforts, the 3 of them, the full code, the epinephrine, simply did not work. Even in witnessed cardiac arrest, survival is about 5%."

Andrea Mitchell - "And Tim Russert's physical condition, his health, his weight - he exercised every day. I know he was coming here right from the treadmill."

Dr. Newman - "His weight was an issue. Weight's something that we all struggle with. Tim struggled with it. And he always said, 'tomorrow! I'm going to start tomorrow, doc. I know what I have to do."

Andrea Mitchell - "Mike Newman, I know you as a friend of Tim's. And I know how hard this is for you. And as his doctor, and how painful this is for everyone connected. And, we just want to thank you for sharing with our viewers, to be as open as possible about what happened here today. It was probably a comfort to people in this bureau to know that he was under your care. And he was working to manage his condition. So thank you."

Dr. Newman - "It's an extraordinary loss. And it's something that, I'm certain, for all of us, we appreciate the uncertainty of our lives."

Andrea Mitchell - "Never more so than tonight. There was no one better, larger, more heroic, more courageous in every aspect of his life - more loving to his family, to his friends, to his employees than my colleague, Timothy J. Russert."

The office where Russert died was that of WRC-TV. It housed the DC bureau of NBC News. He was the bureau chief. According to NBC journalist Brian Williams, Russert's last words were, "What's happening?" spoken in greeting to the editing supervisor Candace Harrington as he passed her in the hallway. He then walked down the hall to the soundproof booth.

As co-workers performed CPR, others called the DC Fire & Rescue, who recorded receiving the call at 1:40 p.m. and dispatched an EMS unit. The unit arrived at 1:44 p.m. As mentioned by Dr. Newman in the transcript of the NBC News Special Report above, paramedics shocked his heart three times. They were trying to stop the chaotic ventricular fibrillation. But the attempts failed.

The EMS transported Russert to Sibley Memorial Hospital. He arrived at 2:23 p.m. and was pronounced dead.

Dr. Newman mentioned Russert's long flight, mentioning the potential of a pulmonary embolus. That's a sudden blockage in an artery of the lung, usually formed by a clot. We define embolus and other terms in the glossary (in the back of this book.) In Russert's case, there was suspicion that the long flight might have caused a clot in the legs, which traveled up to the lungs (a pulmonary embolus).

Russert was the longest-running host of Meet The Press, starting in 1991. He was passionate. His research was extensive. He often found quotes or video clips inconsistent with the current actions of high-profile government guests. A favorite line of his, "these were your words from __ years ago, but now you __." Russert once said, "Our job is that of watchdog… to hold our government accountable to its people."

Inside the left anterior descending artery of Russert's heart, an inflamed, soft plaque ruptured. It ended Russert's TV appearances, voice-overs, research, interviews, and career. It was a critical loss, not only to Russert and his family but to the nation.

In an article on June 17th, a New York Times reporter stated that Russert and his doctors did not know there was a plaque in the arteries of his heart. The doctors "did not realize how severe the disease was because he did not have chest pain or other telltale symptoms that would have justified the kind of invasive tests needed to make a definitive diagnosis. In that sense, his case was sadly typical: more than 50 percent of all men who die of coronary heart disease have no previous symptoms, the American Heart Association says." In another interview, Dr. Newman and Dr. George Bren (Russert's cardiologist) said the autopsy found significant blockages in several coronary arteries (New York Times 2008).

That statement by the New York Times reporter that the doctors did not know Russert had plaque was incorrect. The NBC News Special Report transcript above shows that Russert and his doctors knew about existing plaque ("he had coronary artery disease"). Remember that Russert had a positive Coronary Calcium Score (a sign of coronary heart disease) a decade earlier. But they were surprised by the extent of the disease.

The following year, 2009, was the first year that screening of asymptomatic individuals was recommended by the ACC (American College of Cardiology), The AHA's (American Heart Association) Expert Panel began recommending routine screening of asymptomatic individuals >45 in 2000.

THAT WAS OVER TEN YEARS AGO. WHAT ABOUT NOW?

Has medicine improved much since Russert died? Can we do better in terms of helping patients understand the urgency of their cardiovascular disease? Why do we still hear about heart attacks following negative stress test results?

Why not ask Davie Jones, the lead singer of the Monkees - or game show host Alex Trebek? They both had heart attacks following negative stress tests. You cannot ask Gary Shandling. Like Tim Russert, the heart attack following his negative stress test results killed him.

We have known how to treat this disease effectively for over 50 years. Unfortunately, many physicians today are treating risk factors for disease (Blood Pressure, Cholesterol, etc.) instead of treating the active disease. There is a difference.

Treating atherosclerotic disease and inflammation requires us to monitor its progression (or regression) in order to assess how much more or less aggressive to get in the medical intervention.

Stress tests, which are the primary tool used by cardiologists, help physicians determine whether a surgical (vs. a medical) intervention is warranted. Medical interventions include lifestyle changes and the use of medications, inclusive of pharmaceutical drugs, but also vitamins and supplements. Surgical interventions involve invasive surgical procedures which repair a specific section in need of urgent care.

There are nearly 100,000 miles of vessels in the average adult human body – a stent (a surgical procedure to open a blocked vessel) repairs about 2 inches of that vasculature. It is equivalent to your dentist scraping part of one tooth in your mouth. We do not wish to diminish the importance or value of these surgical interventions. They can be lifesaving when done at the time of a heart attack. But we do want to emphasize a more effective approach for those who have time on their sides.

Medical interventions treat the entire system . . . all 100,000 miles of vessels, whereas surgical interventions are necessarily targeted to a specific area of concern. For those who need surgery, there really are no better options. Most at-risk patients, however, have time to treat their condition medically. These patients can benefit by tools which can help them, and their physicians detect disease earlier in the process, monitor and assess their current disease state in time to treat the disease effectively and prevent further progression.

The tragic story of Tim Russert and many like him, is that they can almost always be prevented. The 'secret sauce' of heart attack and stroke prevention requires monitoring and changing disease treatment using evidence-based medicine. The old model of monitoring and treating just the risk factors for disease does not work as well with heart attack and stroke prevention. This is called secondary prevention. So, instead of just primary prevention (i.e. managing risk factors), secondary prevention (finding and managing early disease) is important in heart attack and stroke prevention. To further clarify this position, let us review some of the tests currently available and how they are utilized.

STRESS TEST RESULT SCENARIOS

There are only four stress test result scenarios:

1. A "false negative" test result - Russert's story was a false negative result. The term "false negative" is in quotation marks because one could debate that the stress test correctly showed good cardiovascular exercise tolerance. But we assume that Russert used his stress test to predict his future risk of experiencing a heart attack or stroke. For that purpose, his stress results were incorrect.

2. A "true positive" - If Russert's stress test had indicated any of a host of problems, it would have resulted as a true positive. Most doctors would have recommended a coronary angiogram (a trip to the catheter lab). The post-mortem indicates Russert had plaque. The cardiologists might have recommended a stent, but it is not likely a stent would have prevented the upcoming heart attack. Studies such as the COURAGE trial indicate that the stent would not have prevented the impending heart attack. (Boden 2007).

3. A false positive - Depending on the studies and definition of false positives, the rates of positive stress tests that are false range from 32.5% to much higher. (Qamruddin 2016) A false positive stress test result frequently leads to a coronary angiogram in a catheter lab. It is fairly common to have atherosclerotic plaque, whether or not it is causing a blockage. It is also common to have that plaque stented.

4. A true negative. - The patient has a negative stress test result and there is no looming heart attack.

Only one of these four test results is a good one, that is the true negative result. When faced with a negative result, we must remember that as many as 15% or more are false negatives like Russert's. Neither of the positive results (true positive and false positive) result in improved patient care (weight loss and other lifestyle and medication treatments). Instead, the positive results usually lead to a trip to the catheter lab and then to a stent or bypass surgery. Stents and bypass surgeries often result in a false sense of security on the part of physicians and their patients.

Why can't we predict heart attacks more accurately? Just what is arterial plaque anyway? How is inflammation related to heart attack and stroke risk or to arterial atherosclerotic plaque?

Over half of all heart attack victims discover they have risk at the point they have a heart attack. High LDL values do not warn over half of those victims; these patients have normal LDL levels. (Bhatt 2015). Over half of the deaths from heart attack and stroke are from sudden cardiac death – meaning these patients had no prior signs or symptoms, like Russert. People that rely on stress tests will continue to be surprised by heart attacks. This is partially due to what stress tests tell us and what they DON'T tell us.

SUDDEN CARDIAC ARREST

Sudden cardiac death is the cause of more natural sudden deaths in the US than anything else. It causes about 325,000 adult deaths in the US each year. It is responsible for over half of all heart disease deaths. (Cleveland Clinic 2019). Sudden cardiac death appears on 13.5% of death certificates in the US each year. One of every 7.4 people in the US will die of sudden cardiac arrest each year. (Benjamin 2018).

Sudden cardiac death is not as unpredictable as most think. Harvard Health explained this over a decade ago: "The perception of sudden cardiac arrest certainly furthered by its name, is that it comes as a bolt out of the blue. A meticulous study by German researchers suggests that it is more like real lightening, which is usually preceded by clouds, wind, and rain." (Harvard Heart Letter 2006).

One of Russert's most significant problems was that he was unaware that he was so close to experiencing a heart attack. There were problems identified in his medical examinations. These issues lead to the stress test and medication adjustments in April. Unfortunately, the stress test results incorrectly indicated that there was no cause for alarm. This contributed to the perception that his problem was neither urgent nor serious, so he relaxed. Had Russert known that he was weeks away from a heart attack, he could have taken measures (like weight loss, and medication adjustments) necessary to reverse his CVC inflammation. Weight loss in patients with CV disease is often lifesaving. We used to think of fat as a harmless energy storage tissue. We know better now.

Fat is an endocrine tissue. It releases chemicals that make the body resistant to insulin, resulting in prediabetes (or insulin resistance) and CV (cardiovascular) inflammation. (Coelho 2013). Dr. Newman spoke to Russert's challenges with weight: "His weight was an issue. His weight was an issue. That is something we all struggle with. Tim struggled with it. And he always said, 'tomorrow! I'm going to start tomorrow, doc. I know what I have to do." Russert was able to discipline himself to exercise, but not to lose weight. He kept promising to do it "tomorrow". Unfortunately, his stress test results incorrectly indicated that there would be time to deal with it later.

This book is about cardiovascular (CV) plaque measurement and risk assessment. CV inflammation causes arterial plaque and ruptured plaque is responsible for the majority of heart attacks and strokes. We begin with a description of CV inflammation, then we describe the commonly used methods of assessing CV plaque and risk (Framingham, stress tests, coronary angiography). Next, we describe other options (Coronary Calcium Score, CIMT, CT Angiogram, ABI, and vascular function testing). Finally, we dive deeper into test characteristics that matter (overutilization, radiation, false positives/negatives).

Physician and patient behaviors are greatly influenced by medical standards committees, so we cover current challenges in the medical standards for CV risk evaluation. We see failure to use CIMT as a major gap in the current healthcare system, so we provide detail on the standards committees' positions on CIMT. We compare the resulting standards to the current science on CIMT. We start and end the book with patient success stories who utilized these technologies. These stories help introduce and demonstrate key concepts about event prevention.

There is a lot of science in this book. It is impossible to write for every level of reader, knowledge, and interest level, but we were anxious to make this book accessible and understandable by everyone, not just your physician. Having said that, we believe this book will also enlighten physicians who have hesitated to use the technologies discussed. We provide hints on sections that can be skipped by those seeking less detail. We also provide a glossary of terms and a bibliography reference tool for those interested in further research.

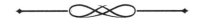

SUMMARY OF THE BOOK

INTENDED AUDIENCE AND PURPOSE

We wrote this book for: Ford's YouTube channel viewers; for those who have family history of heart disease which worries or concerns them, for anyone who has a friend or family adversely affected by a heart attack or stroke, and for those with a heightened interest in heart disease-its etiology and pathophysiology. We also wrote this for physicians seeking evidence-based medical insight they can use in their day-to-day practice, and most of all for patient self-advocates.

Most of those who read this book are people seeking their own medical information. Some are medical science geeks. Some are doctors. There are a lot of CV disease patients seeking explanations and direction on a better way to attack their disease. This book cuts across several of those categories to deal with one of the most significant destructive forces in medicine at this point in history.

Doctors and patients both incorrectly assume that cholesterol and blood pressure tests alone, followed by stress tests, coronary angiograms, and stents/bypasses are the best way to detect and treat heart disease. That incorrect assumption is killing and disabling more people than anything else in the modern and industrialized world.

We are not suggesting these tests should never be used, we are simply showing the obvious, that these tests have not significantly reduced the morbidity and mortality rates of these diseases. We have known how to prevent and treat the disease effectively for nearly 50 years. Unfortunately, the current healthcare system is significantly under-diagnosing those with disease. We must necessarily concern ourselves with evidence-based methods which can more effectively diagnose and monitor efficacy of treatment in order to affect a change on these attack rates.

"Doctor bashing" is not the goal of this book. Although Ford is a physician and Todd is a research doctor - Doctors often have the unenviable position of cleaning up the mess when it is too late - frequently after years of damage to the arteries has already occurred.

On the other hand, doctors do have a leadership role in this space. We can do much better. It is easy to blame the failure to reduce events significantly on financial conspiracy by doctors and hospitals. There may be some of that, to be sure, however, we have found that most physicians want to do the right thing.

Two other actors enter the picture: medical standards committees and insurance companies. We will not discuss insurance companies other than to make this one statement: insurance companies force physicians (via payment policies) to do an hour of prevention in approximately seven minutes. This is an unrealistic expectation, and it is completely untenable if we want to affect change via preventative strategies.

We have a full chapter on medical standards committees. Standards committee members, like doctors and patients, are human. Despite all their excellent work, they are fallible. Their instructions to sit down with the patient and "have a CV risk discussion" have been far too general for a physician who cannot afford to spend more than an average of seven minutes per patient. Also, there are some key medical technologies, like CIMT, which standards committees have failed to recognize and where they have often misinterpreted the available science. We discuss that in detail later in this book.

Most of all, this book was written for patient self-advocates. Until the YouTube channel, more than one third of Ford's practice were doctors and dentists. There are a lot of smart people out there who understand that modern medicine is a "buyer beware" and "buyer must BE aware" environment. It is a challenge to have to learn as much or more about a condition than your physician. However, given the current healthcare environment, it is the best way to avoid life-threatening decisions.

Given the multiple levels of audience sophistication and interest of those who may access this book, we target these disparate audiences at several levels. First, we attempt to describe the current condition in terms of human tragedy and addresses technical misunderstandings that contributed to that outcome.

We provide warnings when the material is about to go into deep detail so that those who maintain a mere parochial interest may skip ahead or use them only as a reference. There is a glossary and bibliography at the end of the book. These are for your ongoing reference and provide those wishing further study into a particular subject a guide on where to find the complete peer-reviewed material. Some may find these the most valuable sections of the book.

WHAT THIS BOOK COVERS

This book provides a view on how to improve the prevention side of cardiovascular medicine by:

1. Changing the current patient care process: Continue to assess patients using Framingham-like risk assessments, (e.g. assessments of risk factors for disease).

2. Adding "nontraditional" risk factors assessment using technologies like CIMT, CAC, CRP/inflammatory testing, gum disease, and others as warranted by the discovery of additional risks); and

3. Improving opportunities for patients to learn what they need to know to prevent their death and disability. This can include recommending excellent strategies for prevention like those outlined by Dr.'s Amy Doneen and Bradly Bale in their book "Beat The Heart Attack Gene", or Dr Robert Superko's book "Before The Heart Attacks". Other books which should be on every heart disease patient's reading list include Dr. Jason Fung's book "The Obesity Code", or Dr. Valter Longo's book "The Longevity Diet". Of course, there are way too many good books on the subject of wellness to mention in this space, but these are a few of our favorites.

4. Avoid tangential and non-contributory tests like nuclear stress testing, coronary angiogram, stents and/or bypass grafts – except when indicated by one of the screening tools above, or when a patient is symptomatic.

This book barely touches on a larger issue: uncovering hidden prediabetes. If we just added two simple, inexpensive, and older tests to the routine preventive assessment of patients, we would revolutionize chronic disease care and prevention. Those two tests are the OGTT (Oral Glucose Tolerance Test) and the Insulin Survey. Descriptions of these tests and their importance are mentioned later in this book. A deeper discussion of these topics is currently planned for in another book. Two excellent books available on this topic include: "Blood Sugar 101", by Jenny Ruhl and The Diabetes Epidemic & You", but Robert Kraft.

These recommendations to change our preventive evaluations are not coming in a vacuum. Experts, task forces, and even medical practice standards bodies have voiced these recommendations before. These suggestions will likely be ignored for a long time by many physicians and their patients. Medicine in the US is vast and comprehensive; it will take a long time to "turn the ship." As the science of CV risk evaluation develops, the standards will change. As the standards change, medical practices will change. Financial incentives do slow the progression of medicine to a safer, better method of CV preventive medicine. Informed patients will hasten the changes. It is a lot to ask a patient to focus on this type of detailed information, but many patients know that medicine is still very much a "buyer-beware" and "buyer BE aware" environment. A few hours spent reading this book can save your life.

WHAT THIS BOOK DOESN'T COVER

This book does not cover many of the CV (cardiovascular) disease management topics. There are already countless books on the countless subtopics involved in medical management of this disease. Despite all those books, too many of us forget this truth; you cannot supplement, medicate, stent, or bypass your way out of a lifestyle problem, or, as another friend of ours put it "There is not a pill made that is more effective than lifestyle choices". (Dr. David Wright)

This book does not even cover all the details of the CV risk assessment. Out of necessity, we introduce the concept of CV inflammation and we cover it in more detail later in this book. An introduction to CV inflammation is required to understand the actual mechanism of heart attack events. However, a basic understanding of that mechanism is required for individuals to understand why stress tests, angiograms, stents, and even bypasses frequently do not work as intended.

This book also does not cover medications, supplements, or many lifestyle/ medical interventions. It does not cover the connections between gum disease and/or stress and CV health. Over half the adults in the US are currently burning their arteries with undiagnosed insulin resistance – but we do not have the space to adequately cover that subject in this book. If this sounds like hyperbole, read on. We touch on it enough to make you wonder if it could be true. Coverage of these other topics would require other books, which may be forthcoming.

A COUPLE OF KEY DEFINITIONS

No book covering improvement in healthcare practice can avoid technical words. We do not attempt to avoid technical words as much as we attempt to explain them. We provide some definitions in the text, but many more appear in a glossary at the back of this book. There is one word we think we should define before going any further: "Cardiovascular". The conflation in this term is a root cause of our failures to deal with chronic diseases, death, and disability. If that sounds like more hyperbole, read on, and think about it.

Cardiovascular (CV) is a conflated term. The roots of the word imply heart and vascular disease. The first half of the term might be a red herring. The real driver or mediator of cardiovascular wellness is arterial health, not just cardio (heart) health. Arterial disease does cause the vast majority of heart disease, and therefore death. However, many are unaware that arterial disease also causes the majority of stroke, kidney, eye disease, and is responsible for high blood pressure. It may be the biggest cause of dementia. In other words, arterial disease is a major contributor to what we now know as chronic disease or aging. The first exposure for many men to the impact and effect of arterial disease occurs when they experience erectile dysfunction.

CV disease is the biggest killer and disabler in the world. Most arterial disease is caused, in turn, by insulin resistance (prediabetes or metabolic syndrome). Many people first notice this as an increase in the size of their belly, which they mistakenly believe is a benign condition; 'the weight gain of middle age'. Although this is not a book about insulin resistance (prediabetes), we cannot neglect it entirely. It is the major cause of arterial disease and dysfunction. This book is about identifying the conditions invoked by inflammation and avoiding the most common mistakes leading to death and disability. Our focus for this book is on medical imaging and assessment of arterial inflammation and heart attack risk.

A BRIEF INTRODUCTION TO INFLAMMATION AND THE METHODS FOR MEASURING PLAQUE/CV RISK

The concluding pages of this chapter introduce CV inflammation and the methods for measuring CV plaque and risk. They summarize the most extensive section of this book, the detailed descriptions of test procedures. For readers that want to skim the book, we recommend reading these brief introductions and then skipping the separate chapters on each specific test for later reference. The specific chapters will be helpful reading when you get a recommendation from your doctors to have one of these tests.

CV INFLAMMATION

Inflammation is the body's response to injury. CV inflammation starts with injury to the delicate lining of the arteries. After that injury, cholesterol and other pathogens seep through the lining. These pathogens, like cholesterol, get stuck in the walls of the artery invoking an immune response. The byproduct of this immune response is inflammation, and eventually the creation of an atherosclerotic lesion called plaque. The immune system recognizes these misplaced pathogens as an injury. The immune system then attacks the pathogen stuck inside the arterial wall. It attempts to dissolve the pathogen using enzymes that liquify it. The next intended step is swallowing the liquid plaque by other specialized immune cells. This is a process called phagocytosis. Samples of these "liquefaction enzymes" and biomarkers include a long list. Here are a few examples: interleukin-1B (IL-1B), Tissue Necrotic Factor (TNF-a) and other inflammation causing cytokines and enzymes. As the cells involved in consuming liquid pathogens complete their process, they dispose of necrotic (dead) material. Incomplete disposal of this necrotic material results in inflamed atherosclerotic plaque lesions. (Meng, 2015). For a more detailed description of CV inflammation, see this book's chapter on Inflammation.

FRAMINGHAM RISK ESTIMATOR

Doctors first estimate CV risk by listing key risk factors like age, gender, smoking & diabetes status. These risk factors have each been shown to increase a person's lifetime risk of cardiovascular disease independently. Family history is used as a proxy for genetic status. This too is another source of error. Ford has trained and worked in genetic labs. Family history often ignores the fact that people can get uncommonly expressed genes in their family and sometimes there are unknown "family members" contributing unrecognized genes to the pool. Lab values such as cholesterol and diabetes status are also used if available. Based on this information, estimates of CV risk are developed. These risk factors, (collectively referred to as the Framingham Risk estimator), and other risk prediction models, are usually used to develop key CV risk management recommendations. As we will see later, problems with the Framingham risk estimator lead to the common practice of statin over-prescription.

STRESS TESTS

The stress test is a procedure used to measure heart function during physical activity. It typically involves stimulation of the heart's response to exercise using a treadmill, exercise bike, or drugs. They measure cardiac conditioning, usually via ultrasound, electrical signal monitoring and other combinations of technologies. It is important to understand, however, that none of these technologies measure plaque or heart attack risk. When used to predict heart attack risk, the positive and negative test results are often false, or incorrect. Medical researchers have done a lot to improve stress tests, trying multiple methods to assess heart function during the test. The most popular version of the stress test, by far, is the nuclear stress test with over 8 million tests completed each year in the US alone. The nuclear stress testing involves the injection of a radioactive dye which facilitates imaging, making it easier to see and measure cardiac conditioning.

Stress tests are examples of flow studies. The term "flow study" means that blood flow is measured, but not plaque. It is important to understand that a ruptured plaque can cause a blockage of blood flow very quickly – but the plaque themselves rarely cause blockage UNTIL they rupture.

Measuring blood flow is like measuring the volume of water coming through a garden hose. If the garden hose is not kinked, the water flows smoothly through the hose at some predictable rate. Only when the hose is kinked or blocked by more than 50% does the velocity of the water change – demonstrated by the water spraying out the end of the hose. The same can be said of all tests which measure blood flow. Because these studies only see changes in velocity of the blood flow resulting from a blocked or partially blocked vessel, these flow studies create significant diagnostic problems.

Stress tests do not detect plaque until there is ≥ 50%- occlusion (or blockage) of blood flow in the artery. (Falk, 1995) This is why Russert and hundreds of thousands of others have died after receiving recent negative stress test results. Even though they had significant amounts of plaque in their arteries, there was not enough plaque to cause a blockage ≥ 50% of blood flow at the time of their exam. For most heart attack victims, there is little or no blockage of their artery minutes before their heart attack or stroke.

Blockage occurs when the plaque breaks off and lodges up or downstream or a clot is formed while trying to heal the ruptured plaque lesion, and the clot breaks off and lodges up or downstream of its origin with a liquid plaque release.

Russert's case is endemic and prevalent in the majority of heart attack and stroke victims; 86% of the heart attacks occur in people with less than 70% occlusion (blockage of blood flow) in their arteries and 68% of heart attacks occur in people with less than 50% occlusion. (Falk 1995). This means that for most of the heart attack and stroke victims in the US – they do not have any significant blockage which could be detected by ANY flow study . . . until their plaque ruptured . . . suddenly and spontaneously . . . at which time they very quickly formed a blockage which resulted in a clinical event.

For almost a decade, most medical standards committees have discouraged the current high rates of stress (flow) testing. The following governing bodies have provided guidelines advising against stress tests in low risk, asymptomatic (without signs or symptoms) individuals (Choosing Wisely®, "Annual EKGs for Low-risk Patients," AAFP News, https://www.aafp.org/patient-care/clinical-recommendations/all/cw-ekg.html):

- The US Preventive Services Task Force (Moyer, 2012);
- The American Academy of Family Physicians (AAFP, 2012);
- The American College of Cardiology (Greenland P, 2010);
- The American Heart Association (Hendel RC, 2009).

CORONARY ANGIOGRAMS

A coronary angiogram is a procedure where radioactive dye is injected into the heart's arteries to facilitate or enhance an Xray image. The injection is usually administered using a catheter which is inserted into the femoral artery at the groin and threaded up through the aorta to the heart. Other names for this test include coronary artery angiogram, cath angiogram, heart catheterization, and cardiac cath.

We mentioned that many stress tests result in trips to the catheter lab. Many catheter lab procedures result in the additional procedure of a stent placement or even a bypass graft. A common practice, at facilities where these procedures are performed, involves getting consent for a stent and even a bypass graft any time a catheter angiogram is administered. The progression from stress test to catheter angiogram to stent is a tragically common triad in cardiology. This practice of unnecessary and automatic escalation of procedures costs the American healthcare system billions of dollars each year.

CTA (Computerized Tomography Angiogram)

The Computerized Tomography Angiogram is a procedure which uses radioactive dye or contrast material, injected into the veins of the arm, to facilitate the imaging of plaque and the anatomy of the coronary arteries using an intravenous Xray and CT imaging. Recent studies indicate this could bring much clarity to the usual stress test practices. There has been a rapid "learning curve," resulting in more opportunities for the use of CTA. More frequent use of the latest equipment could reduce the amount of unnecessary patient radiation exposure.

CORONARY CALCIUM SCORE

The Coronary Calcium Score measures calcium in the arteries of the heart using radiated CT imaging. The presence of any calcium indicates there is plaque in these arteries. This test is easily accessible, inexpensive, and well standardized. It is a great screening tool. It is not a good test for monitoring progress or change. We describe why in the chapter on the Coronary Calcium Score.

Carotid Intima-Media Thickness Testing (CIMT)

The Carotid Intima-Media Thickness (CIMT) is the only non-invasive test that measures arterial inflammation and plaque. That statement is worth repeating. Remember, inflammation and plaque cause heart attacks. The CIMT is the only non-invasive test that measures arterial inflammation and plaque. It is important to differentiate this from tests which simply estimate a patient's risk of inflammation and/or plaque development via arterial blood flow restriction. CIMT is a direct measure of how much or how little inflammation and/or plaque one has inside their arteries. Measurement is done in the arteries of the neck or groin using ultrasound technology and software analytics. Ultrasound is a technology which uses sound waves. There is no use of radiation or contrast material into the patient's arteries for this test – only sound waves. CIMT is not expensive. There is no disrobing required for a carotid IMT, and only minimal disrobing required for a femoral artery IMT exam. CIMT is also the only test that provides critical information on the characterization of the plaque (e.g. whether plaque is soft and dangerous, heterogenous or echogenic and healed). Given all these advantages, why has CIMT been ignored? CIMT suffers from a lack of standardization. We discuss this disadvantage in detail. We also discuss how it has been overcome.

ABI (Ankle Brachial Index)

An Ankle Brachial Index is a comparison of the ankle and arm blood pressures. If the ankle pressure is low compared to the arm, this implies peripheral disease in the arteries between the heart and ankle, which could include plaque or flow disruption. This test is simple in concept but also suffers from standardization and quality failures. Like the CIMT, the ABI requires robust quality systems.

VASCULAR FUNCTION TESTING

These tests measure the functional abilities of the arteries such as expansion (dilation) and constriction in response to challenges. Vascular function testing can measure the artery's inherent elasticity, but also a phenomenon known as post occlusive reactive hyperemia, which is the body and artery's ability to get back to homeostasis following a blockage in the blood vessel. Vascular dysfunction is one of the earliest signs of vascular disease. Like the CIMT and ABI, these tests can be helpful, but require advanced quality systems to be reliable.

TEST CHARACTERISTICS AND PROBLEMS

The section of the book following the detailed description of each test goes into general CV testing problems. These sections provide more detail on overutilization, radiation, sensitivity/specificity and false test results. Below is a summary of some of the important considerations which are more completely addressed in subsequent sections of this book.

A. Drivers of Overutilization: Stress tests, catheter labs, angiograms, and stents/grafts are overused, often for financial reasons. Not all overutilization is related to just financial motives. Patients have limited access to information about their arterial health. Making the best choice about optimal testing requires an understanding of the variables contributing to some physician's suboptimal recommendations.

B. Radiation: The triad mentioned above (stress tests, catheter angiography, and stenting) deliver significant radiation. Radiation cancer risk, resulting from these procedures, is usually considered minimal compared to the risk for heart attack or stroke. However, when repeated procedures or combinations of procedures are used, or when these procedures are conducted on younger aged patients, this is not always the case.

C. Test characteristics: Sensitivity and specificity are technical terms that describe the value of screening tests. In short, the term Sensitivity refers to the ability of a test to correctly identify those with a disease (the true positive rate). While Specificity refers to the ability of a test to correctly identify those without the disease (the true negative rate). Any valid and useful test must balance the statistical demands of these two important considerations. The statistics which describe this methodology are beyond the scope of this book. There is enough discussion of the topic to demonstrate why so many false positive and false negative test results are largely ignored.

CHRONIC DISEASE MODELS: CUT POINTS TURN PEOPLE INTO PATIENTS

The diagnosis of coronary artery disease begins with a dilemma. There is no consensus on how much plaque is required for a diagnosis of this disease. (Arbab-Zadeh, 2012). Most adults (and even many teens) have plaque in their coronary arteries, yet they appear healthy. (Nemetz PN, 2008) (Tuzcu EM, 2001) Medical scientists have been aware of the presence of plaque in apparently healthy people for decades. Unlike other diseases such as cancers or infections, the diagnosis of CV disease is not categorical. As it relates to CV disease, the presence or absence of a condition is neither absolute nor directive until it becomes symptomatic. We have therefore imposed a model using a quantitative cut point.

A cut point is a subjective level which expresses the point at which a disease process becomes remarkable. Patients are scored on the amount of inflammation or plaque relative to others ("normals"). If there is more than a certain amount of plaque, a diagnosis is given, and the person becomes a patient. This subjective categorical approach is the same used in other chronic diseases like diabetes and high blood pressure. (Kraft, 2008) (Casey DE, 2019)

Defining the cut points that turn these people into patients is an endless and expensive process. The resulting confusion leaves a wake of unnecessary disease, disability, and death.

Diabetes expert panels chose round numbers (100 for normal, 200 for diabetes). (ADA, 2018) People with blood sugars in between those two 'cut points' are confused about whether they have the disease or not. Many experts have assumed that the cut point for defining plaque as a disease should be the point at which it obstructs blood flow. (Arbab-Zadeh, 2012) It is time to question these assumptions as they have resulted in CV disease death exceeding the next 3 leading causes of disease combined. Redefining these assumptions moves us toward a new definition of CV disease and even aging. More importantly, redefining these cut points enables us to treat the disease medically and in time to avoid an escalated and often emergency surgical intervention, unnecessary disability, or death.

WORN OUT ASSUMPTIONS IN CV DISEASE

We rely on assumptions. We then test these assumptions for validity. In time, they improve our efficiency. Sometimes, however, they create more harm than good. For example, stress tests are over-utilized in part because of the assumption that CV exercise conditioning is the same as heart attack risk abatement and should therefore be assessed. There is some correlation between conditioning and heart attack risk, but there is a better way. It starts with giving up 2 other worn-out assumptions:

1. The assumption that high LDL is the major risk factor for heart attack and stroke; and

2. The assumption that heart attacks happen the same way that hair clogs the shower drain; by slowly building up on the inside of the "pipe" to choke off the flow.

Upon giving up those assumptions, new paradigms need to take their place. These new paradigms require understanding the actual mechanism or pathophysiology of heart attacks. The pathophysiology of heart disease which results in a heart attack, involves a progression in the arterial walls from inflammation to plaque formation, to plaque rupture and release of enzymes into the blood stream which lead to blood clot formation and blockage of blood flow.

Heart attacks are rarely gradual and predictable, like a shower drain clogging with increasing hair deposits. Heart attacks most often occur suddenly, with little or no warning. This is because plaques also rupture suddenly and without much warning. We can visually witness this progression using ultrasound and other technologies which allow us to see the inside of the arterial wall.

These new paradigms fit the facts; risk builds with the disease until an event (heart attack) occurs. Although we still cannot predict the exact timing of a heart attack or stroke, we can do much better at assessing where a patient is along the pathophysiological pathway. Just as storms are strongly correlated with lightning, so too CV inflammation and soft plaque formation are strongly correlated to heart attack and stroke. The next logical step then, is the measurement of CV inflammation and plaque. With better knowledge of these "metabolic storms" (inflammation and plaque formation), risk management improves.

In the following pages of this section, we will describe the real mechanism for heart attacks. Then we will delve deeper into the detail of the processes that lead to inflammation and CV plaque formation. Finally, we will provide some information on CV inflammation testing. The focus of the rest of the book is on better inflammation assessment, plaque measurement, and plaque characterization.

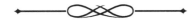

CARDIOVASCULAR DISEASE

ESSENTIAL BACKGROUND INFORMATION:

CV INFLAMMATION. WHAT IS IT? HOW DO WE MEASURE IT?

Atherosclerosis is like the formation of acne inside the walls of the artery. The description of Russert's arteries at autopsy was analogous to a bad case of facial acne. Most of us assume that plaque lines the inside space (lumen) of an artery like hair lining the inside of a shower drain where the water flows. That assumption is incorrect. We will describe why that is important to know later.

Plaque formation occurs between layers of the artery walls (the intima and media layers). As cholesterol or other pathogens penetrate the inner wall or lining of the artery, it attracts the body's immune cells (monocytes) to the wall surface. These cells are then converted to pathogen destroying cells (macrophages) where they begin to attack these pathogens in a similar manner to how they attack a virus or bacteria.

The macrophages essentially consume these pathogens until they are destroyed. The byproduct of this process are foam cells and fatty streaks which are inflammatory. Also, some of the macrophages attract cytokines and other inflammatory enzymes which cause additional inflammation in the arterial wall. Eventually, the accumulation of cellular waste or necrotic material (the white pussy stuff you would see in a facial acne lesion) grows inside the arterial wall and forms a lesion. These lesions attract other cells which weaken the arterial wall, making the lesion more likely to rupture. The combination of necrotic core material forming an atherosclerotic lesion, combined with the attraction and release of cytokines and enzymes which weaken the arterial wall and lead to clot formation work together to cause a plaque erosion or rupture. This rupture leads to a cascade of activities that very often result in the formation of a thrombus or blood clot which often blocks the blood flow entirely. (Meng, 2015)

Large clots can block blood flow to the tissue, starving it of oxygen and killing it. When the oxygen-starved tissue is in the heart, the result is a heart attack. When the oxygen-starved tissue is in the brain, the result is a stroke. Dying heart tissue creates chaotic heartbeats (fibrillation). Without coordinated beats, the pump function of the heart disappears. Blood stops flowing, leading to a loss of consciousness, followed by death.

The rest of this appendix describes the cellular biology and testing for CV inflammation. It is written for medical doctors, patients with more than a passing interest in pathophysiology, and biology geeks. If your goal is simply a better understanding of plaque measurement, you might consider skipping it.

INFLAMMATION AND PLAQUE DEVELOPMENT

The Walls or Layers or the Artery

The intima is a thin lining of the artery wall which is generally believed to include a single-cell layer called the endothelium. The endothelium is the largest organ in the body. It lines all 100,000 miles of vasculature in adults, and it lines every other organ in the body.

The endothelium provides a slick coating to support blood flow. It also provides an interface for cellular metabolism. Cells in the body tissues exchange oxygen, energy sources, and metabolites for carbon dioxide and waste products.

The media is the smooth muscular layer of the artery walls. This layer provides strength and structural integrity and provides the gentle elastic motion of contraction and relaxation required to pump blood through the body. Its main function is to regulate the caliber of the blood vessels. Excessive vasoconstriction (squeezing of the muscular walls of arteries) leads to high blood pressure, while excessive vasodilation leads to low blood pressure.

The final layer is the tunica adventitia. This is the hard-white sinewy layer composed mostly of collagenous and elastic fibers. The adventitia provides a limiting barrier and holds the rest of the arterial wall together. Without the adventitia layer, arteries would disintegrate under pressure.

CAN THE PRESENCE OF INFLAMMATION PROVIDE A MORE URGENT WARNING?

Inflammation provides an opportunity for an earlier and less urgent warning of impending heart attack. If we can warn patients that their arteries are currently inflamed, they can better understand the importance of the need to cool those arteries back to their normal state of homeostasis. Rudolf Virchow described arterial inflammation over 150 years ago (Virchow, 1856).

Virchow was well known as the father of two fields of medicine, pathology, and social medicine. Why were his findings of arterial inflammation ignored for over 100 years? Perhaps it was the discovery that most arterial plaque contains oxidized LDL cholesterol. The past 60 years have witnessed a misdirected focus on cholesterol. Many are blaming that on Ancel Keys. (Carroll, April 15, 2016). It is likely the following fact contributed to Ancel Keys' red herring; the primary ingredient of arterial plaque is cholesterol.

Data from the 1990s began to indicate that inflammation, as measured by high-sensitivity C-reactive protein (hs-CRP or CRP for purposes of this book) or interleukin I (IL)-6, was strongly associated with future vascular events, independent of the usual risk factors. (Berk, 1990) and (Liuzzo G, 1994). By 1997, Paul Ridker and others provided compelling data in the Physicians' Health Study. Ridker and others demonstrated elevated hs-CRP levels in healthy subjects in advance of first-ever vascular events. (Ridker PM, 1997).

Cardiovascular inflammation can be a critical warning of imminent danger. Although current US medical standards give hsCRP a minor recommendation (class IIb), committees are too conflicted to mount a coordinated response (Ridker PM, 2015). Part of this hesitancy may be tied to hsCRP's lack of specificity. hsCRP levels are likely to spike for infections like the common cold, or the flu, or arthritis. This does not render it useless in any way – it just means that users need to understand what they are looking at when they see an elevated hsCRP test result. One of the answers could be arterial wall inflammation. Too few doctors use this important bio-monitor and too few patients are aware of it.

Michael Newman ordered the hsCRP on Tim Russert. So why didn't it show inflammation? Similar to the stress test, the hsCRP test is known for false positives and negatives. This is why we recommend multiple tests which look for CV inflammation.

Brad Bale and Amy Doneen have been teaching methods of CV risk assessment for nearly two decades. In 2014, they published a book titled BEAT THE HEART ATTACK GENE. (Bale B, 2014). Physicians and non-physicians alike have read the book. It provides many examples of better ways to detect and manage heart attack & stroke risk.

SOFT PLAQUE RUPTURE LEADS TO CLOT FORMATION

The acne-like lesions lining the walls of Russert's arteries in the autopsy were atherosclerotic plaques. One of those "pimples" ruptured, spewing its contents into the bloodstream. The inflammatory components of that soft plaque activated the platelets in the blood which caused the blood to form a clot.

The clot blocked the arteries providing blood and therefore oxygen to the muscle in Russert's heart. Finally, this oxygen-starved heart muscle created a chaotic rhythm known as ventricular fibrillation. That fibrillation spread to the rest of the heart, resulting in a loss of coordinated pumping function. Blood flow to Russert's body stopped. When blood flow to his brain ceased, Russert lost consciousness. He never woke up.

This same tragedy still occurs every 76 seconds in the US. Heart attacks occur every 38 seconds — half result in sudden death.

Below is an explanation of what probably happened to Russert's arteries leading up to this event.

INFLAMMATION CONTINUED: INJURY TO THE GLYCOCALYX

Ironically, the immune system creates inflammation while working to protect and heal the body. The immune system begins the body's process of injury repair. First, it kills, digests, and removes pathogens (outside organisms that have the potential to cause disease or harm to the body – like bacteria or viruses). The immune system does the same to body tissues if it does not recognize them, or if they are in the wrong locations. Regarding CV inflammation, the artery wall is taking friendly fire from the body's own immune system.

Other body parts can take this friendly fire from the immune system. In the case of rheumatoid arthritis, the immune system attacks joint tissue. With lupus, antibodies to the cell's nucleus indicate another internal target of the immune system attack. Hashimoto's thyroiditis and inflammatory bowel disease are inflammatory, as well. In the case of Hashimoto's disease, the thyroid gland and intestines are the targets. Most of these inflammatory diseases, such as rheumatoid arthritis, also increase heart attack risk.

As we mentioned, one of the most common drivers of heart attack & stroke risk is prediabetes (also called insulin resistance or metabolic syndrome). For this book, we will abbreviate using IR for Insulin Resistance. IR is associated with aging or unhealthy fat stores. It dramatically increases the growth rate of plaque within the artery walls.

The CDC said in 2017 there were over 84 million adults in the US with IR (prediabetes) and 90% of the victims do not know it. (CDC, July 18, 2017). The year before, UCLA reported that over half of all adult Californians have this disease. (Babey SH, 2016). Their estimates were conservative. These estimates were based on fasting glucose and Hemoglobin A1c. Both tests (fasting glucose and HgA1c) have high false-negative rates, even when used together. (Kraft, 2008).

INFLAMMATION INJURES THE ENDOTHELIUM

Inflammation starts with damage to the intima, the thin outer lining of the artery. The point of origin of this injury is damage to the endothelial wall. The cells of the endothelium are permeable. This means other cells (monocytes, cholesterol esters, etc) can slip through and penetrate the wall of the artery. This is important because the artery is a live tissue. Like other live tissues in the body, it needs nourishment in the form of oxygen, and energy. The problem comes when a pathogen (a disease-causing entity) penetrates this wall and gets trapped. There are many chemical and other reasons which lead to lipids and other pathogens to become stuck or trapped in the wall of the artery.

THE GLYCOCALYX

One of the biggest weak spots of the intima appears to be the glycocalyx. The glycocalyx is a part of the intima (or endothelium lining the artery wall). The inside surface of the intima consists of hair-like projections made mostly of sugars and some protein. These hair-like projections appear to be the major area of metabolic activity. This glycocalyx is similar to the marshlands, where the major biologic activity occurs at the grassy intersection of land and water.

The glycocalyx is the location where oxygen and carbon dioxide are exchanged. It is also where other cell inputs and wastes are exchanged. When these pathogens present inside the wall of the artery, they attract a different class of immune cell and activate the body's natural immune response. This targets these cells for destruction, or consumption by the body's immune cells.

The destruction of these cells triggers a cascade response which attracts inflammation causing enzymes and cytokines like TNF and Interleukins (IL). The combination of triggered responses results in the oxidation of lipids (cholesterol).

The body's immune system destroys these lipids and other cells which leads to deposition of foam cells, other necrotic material, and the formation of fatty streaks inside the arterial wall. This necrotic (dead) or waste material precipitated by this process results in additional inflammation. Left unchecked, this process will eventually lead to the formation of atherosclerotic plaque lesions.

Simultaneous to this inflammatory process, additional cells, enzymes, and cytokines are attracted to the area which weaken the wall of the artery and specifically the thin fibrous cap that prevents this necrotic material from seeping into the body's blood stream.

Over time, the plaques rupture or erode much like an acne pimple. This happens both from the shear stress of the blood hitting the lesion 24 hours each day, and from the weakening of the arterial wall from the newly attracted enzymes, which are also trapped inside the wall of this lesion.

Once the plaque erodes or ruptures, additional enzymes are released into the blood stream, some of which activate the platelets of the blood and tell them to form a scab or a thrombus (a blood clot). Remember, this is the body's natural defense to injury – and when we puncture our skin, we want those platelets to activate to form a protective scab over the injured area. Unfortunately, as it relates to an injury on the inside wall of our arteries, these scabs (or thrombi) are extremely dangerous. If not dissolved, they can break off the original site and get pushed into the smaller vessels leading to the brain or heart causing a blockage. They can also grow so large that blood flow is stopped completely. (Meng, 2015)

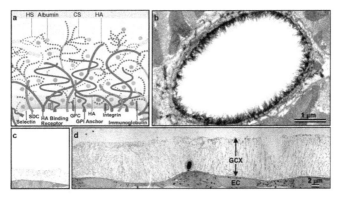

The glycocalyx of the endothelium (or intima) provides increased surface area for the exchange of oxygen, energy, and cell waste products. When the endothelium is injured, it allows LDL to pass through the intima and interact with more free radicals which leads to the LDL molecule becoming oxidized.

Oxidized LDL attracts the body's immune cells to begin the cell destruction process (phagocytosis). Until 2019, medical scientists incorrectly assumed that inflammation created holes in the intima. Philip Shaul's team at UT Southwestern in Dallas demonstrated that it is not holes in the intima, it is a process called transcytosis. Given the fact that cyto means cell, you might guess that it means the LDL and other plaque components are transported through the intima cell. That would be correct; oxLDL is transported directly through the intima cell. (Huang L., 2019)

The oxidized LDL gets stuck in the space between the intima and media layer leading to inflammation and arterial plaque formation. The term IMT stands for "Intima-Media Thickness." Which refers to the net effect of this process to the wall of the artery (e.g. the Intima and Media layers of the artery).

Figure A, in the image on page 45, is a representation of the glycocalyx, showing some of its biological components. Figure B shows a larger picture of the artery wall, using a STORM method microscopy. Figure C shows an injured, thin glycocalyx. Figure D shows a healthy, thicker glycocalyx. (Oshima K, 2017)

Cardiovascular inflammation starts with an injury to the endothelium. High blood sugar, high insulin, or smoking by-products, and other pathogens injure the endothelium. These inflammatory agents make it easier for pathogens like cholesterol to penetrate and get trapped inside the arterial wall.

When the endothelial wall is damaged, LDL and other pathogens pass through the intima layer. (LDL stands for Low-Density Lipoprotein. Many call LDL "bad cholesterol" because it is the primary component of plaque). The MACR test for CV inflammation tests for intimal injury by measuring these injured cells as they pass through the kidney filters.

WHAT IS THE IMMUNE SYSTEM'S "FRIENDLY FIRE"?

When the LDL particles get trapped in the intima-media space, immune cells discover the problem and go into action. Different families of immune cells are involved: monocytes, macrophages, macrocytes, foam cells (a type of macrophage that are attracted to fatty deposits on blood vessel walls), dendric cells, mast cells, and neutrophils.

Monocytes, one family of white cells, pass from the blood through the intima layer to begin work attacking these pathogens. As monocytes move through the intima, they convert into active macrophages (a dynamic version of monocytes).

The macrophages then begin releasing enzymes. The enzymes break down the particles in the arterial wall. The release of enzymes and related cells and molecules in the wall of the artery causes inflammation and soft, liquid plaque.

If the cap of the plaque erodes or ruptures, it releases the liquid plaque (the necrotic white sticky substance very similar to the substance inside a facial acne pimple) into the bloodstream. Liquid plaque can cause blood to clot. If this happens and a large clot forms, it can cause a heart attack or stroke by flowing to an artery in the heart, or brain (respectively) lodging there and blocking the blood supply to tissue up or downstream. (Swirski FK, 2013).

OXIDATION AND INFLAMMATION

Oxidation is a significant driver of the inflammatory process. The decades-long focus on supplements and antioxidants comes from the recognition of oxidation's role in aging. Oxidation gives species such as humans significant advantages in terms of energy. We can extract 36 units of energy from a glucose molecule. That compares to only six energy units derived by more primitive species such as yeast.

The human ability to transport and use oxygen gives us extra power. In return, this oxygen metabolism exacts a toll of increased oxidation. Oxidation is the essential force described in one of the most popular theories of aging – the mitochondrial theory.

In the mitochondrial theory of aging, the furnaces of the cell (mitochondria) slowly decline due to chronic oxidation damage. Your local mechanic calls oxidation "rust "(at least when iron is involved).

Oxidized LDL is much more likely to pass through the injured intima cells. That gives rise to one of our blood tests for the inflammation process. We can test blood for oxLDL (oxidized LDL). This test measures the concentration of oxLDL per unit of blood. The higher the concentration, the more likely one is to have CV disease.

CELLULAR COMPONENTS OF INFLAMMATION

Inflammation is simply the immune system's response to any damage in the body. Once immune cells find their way to the location of plaque, they begin to release enzymes that destroy (liquify, or consume) the oxLDL and other pathogens. Other chemicals are released as well. These other chemicals attract more immune cells to the area of inflammation. These are called cytokines (cyto means "cell," and kines means "attractants").

We mentioned several families of immune cells and a couple of types of chemicals. Inflammation is a complicated process. We will not get any more detailed in terms of the cells and other ingredients in this book, but hopefully we have provided a good overview. Similar processes are involved in the inflammatory stages of facial acne. This is why the analogy of acne within the lining of Russert's arteries fits so well.

As the inflammatory process continues, a pool of liquid material forms. This pool consists of immune cells, cytokines, debris, and other types of necrotic or dead material formed by the immune processes. That pool of materials grows to become soft plaque. The soft plaque includes proteins, oxLDL, glycoproteins, etc. and the necrotic byproduct of pathogenic cell destruction. The material in an atherosclerotic plaque is remarkably similar to the material in that sticky white substance found inside a large facial acne lesion. Some of these components can signal blood to clot. (For the technical geeks, one example is tissue factor, a glycoprotein, also called "factor X." It is an enzyme, part of the cytokine receptor class II.)

Over time, a calcific cap forms over these liquid plaque pools. If the cap breaks, the plaque ruptures and releases the pool of materials contained in the soft plaque into the bloodstream. Also, this necrotic material inside the wall of the artery attracts other enzymes which weaken the outer layers of the wall – and the thin fibrous cap which encapsulates or prevents that white sticky material from being released into the blood stream. Once this wall is compromised, it releases all or much of that material into the blood stream. Some of that material activates the platelets in the blood and instructs them to form a clot or protective scab on the wall of the artery. If the blood clot (embolus) is big enough, or it breaks off (as they often do) they can be pushed to the heart, which causes a heart attack. If the plaque or subsequent thrombus is large enough and goes to the brain, it results in a stroke.

This is the sequence of events that killed Russert. This sequence of events causes a heart attack every 38 seconds in the US. Half of those heart attacks result in sudden death. This process (CV inflammation, plaque rupture, clot formation, and artery blockage) is the most common killer and disabler of humans in the world. Heart attacks and strokes cause a full third of the deaths in the US (38% of the deaths each year in women). Most of those are related to the rupture of an atherosclerotic plaque.

Why then, are most CV events perceived to be unpredictable? This is because we can't predict the rupture of a fibrous cap which protects the inflamed plaque material using stress tests and angiograms. Fortunately, we can now detect and measure inflammation through blood tests and simple artery scans (CIMT).

We have methods to show whether arterial plaque is soft, and liquid filled, or hard as a rock and healed (CIMT). Medical standards do not currently include many of these processes in their assessment recommendations – or they give them a 'luke-warm' recommendation. Again, consider whether you want to go into the level of detail in the subsequent sections of this book, or use it for later reference.

THE INFLAMMATION PANEL LAB TESTS

There is no single definitive test for CV inflammation. There are, however, panels (combinations of tests) that help us measure the processes described above. The CV inflammation panel below is from Cleveland Heart Lab, now owned by Quest Labs. They include CRP, MACR, Lp- PLA2, and MPO. It is important to understand the analytes in these panels and their relationship to the inflammatory process if we are to use them effectively.

CRP (C REACTIVE PROTEIN)

CRP is a protein made by the liver in response to multiple inflammatory challenges. When the body fights inflammation, the liver makes CRP. This includes inflammation within the walls of the arteries. Although some researchers get a CRP analysis done alone in studies, we do not recommend using it alone for an individual patient assessment. There are simply too many false positives and negatives to rely on CRP alone for personalized CV care. For example, some studies have shown that two days after even just a flu shot, two-thirds of us will have an elevated CRP. Consider including the other inflammatory tests listed below.

MACR (MICRO ALBUMIN CREATININE RATIO)

Another test, MACR (microalbumin/creatinine ratio) measures the amount of the protein (Albumin) in the urine. There are about 1 million microscopic filters in each kidney. They filter waste materials from the blood into the urine. The membranes in those filters consist of the intima or lining of the arteries. Usually, the intima membrane retains proteins such as Albumin. If the intima is damaged, Albumin leaks into the urine. As we mentioned earlier, damaged intima also leaks LDL. So, if albumin is leaking into the urine, LDL is likely leaking into the arterial wall.

LP-PLA2

Monocytes slip through the endothelium and into the intima-media space. When these monocytes become activated, they transition into slightly different cell types called macrophages. Macrophages continue to grow and they eventually become scavengers – looking for pathogenic material to destroy and consume. These cells then join other activated macrophages, forming foam cells and fatty streaks. As this process continues, these cells release enzymes, including Lp-PLA2, which is used to destroy and digest cellular trash. Since these enzymes only appear when the cell-destruction process is active, the higher the concentration of Lp-PLA2, the higher the likelihood a patient is fighting active atherosclerotic disease.

MPO (MYELOPEROXIDASE)

Other types of immune cells called polymorphs or neutrophils arrive at the site of CV inflammation as well. They do the same thing as monocytes. The neutrophils release enzymes (myeloperoxidase or MPO).

Lab tests can demonstrate Lp-Pla2 and MPO in the blood. They allow measurement of the inflammatory process inside the wall of the artery. These neutrophils are specific to the inflammatory process within the arterial wall, so they are better (more specific to CV disease) than some of the other tests for inflammation.

INTERLEUKIN 6 (IL6)

Another example of these additional tests is Interleukin 6 (IL6). Interleukins are pro-inflammatory cytokines and anti-inflammatory myokines. Interleukin is a protein which is produced by various cells in the body. It is nearly always elevated with CV diseases but can also be elevated with other infections or autoimmune disorders – so it must be taken into consideration with the other markers/tests for CV disease and inflammation. A more in-depth description of inflammation biomarkers and testing is beyond the scope of this book, but hopefully these brief descriptions will be helpful.

CHOLESTEROL VS. INFLAMMATION

Where does all this leave cholesterol? As we mentioned earlier, oxidized LDL and a protein carrier, APO B (Apolipoprotein B) are the primary atherogenic components of plaque and one of the reasons for the term "bad" cholesterol. (Shapiro, 2017). Preventive standards are slowly de-emphasizing LDL and focusing more on a generalized risk assessment including inflammation assessment. The ACC/ADA prevention standard now gives a moderate (IIb) value to hsCRP.

There is also growing acknowledgement of newer methods of plaque detection, such as the Coronary Calcium Score. It is still too early for the standards changes we predict for CT angiography and CIMT, but we expect to see changes forthcoming. Standards processes take decades to make a significant change (see the section on the medical standards process).

FAMILIAL HYPERCHOLESTEROLEMIA- AN INDICATOR OF THE RELATIVE IMPORTANCE OF LDL?

FH (Familial Hypercholesterolemia) is a genetic variant that results in the production of high levels of LDL (above 200). FH can help us understand the relative importance of LDL among heart attack and stroke risks. FH is a genetic disorder resulting in LDL levels much higher than average. FH happens in about 1 in 200 humans. It is significantly underdiagnosed; far fewer than 1 in 200 have a diagnosis. Most families with FH remain undiagnosed and unaware of their condition. If LDL were the most potent driver of heart attacks, most families would be aware because more family members would die younger. This happens with homozygous FH (a severe form of FH involving disease genes from both parents).

Awareness of aging as a risk factor for CV disease is far more common than is assessment of FH. This is because age is such a strong risk factor in the US. The same applies to full-blown diabetes. As mentioned before, prediabetes is a significant risk factor for CV events. As prediabetes becomes more widely recognized, the association with CV disease will become more well-known and better understood.

CHOLESTEROL MANAGEMENT STANDARDS

LDL, HDL, and other forms of cholesterol in the blood are also called "lipids." The terms lipid means fat or oil. Medical standards committees previously recommended levels of LDL cholesterol below 100. Now they recommend levels below 70. FH should be considered when a patient has ever had an LDL of 180 or higher.

Genetic testing, although imperfect, is a consideration for these FH individuals. There are about 2000 genetic variations that can result in FH, and genetic testing covers only a few. Those few genetic variations account for over 80% of all FH cases. A positive test result for FH does not just help us to treat the patient more effectively. Knowledge of an FH gene in the family helps other family members understand the need for CV risk awareness and treatment.

FH risk is usually easily managed. The risk is more of a decreased capacity to manage other risks, such as smoking or prediabetes. If LDL were the most critical driver of heart attacks, FH risk would not be as easily managed.

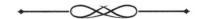

CARDIOVASCULAR PLAQUE & INFLAMMATION

THE REAL MECHANISM OF HEART ATTACKS

Atherosclerosis means scarring of the arteries. From a more practical perspective, having atherosclerosis means you have active disease and plaque in your arteries. The term comes from the Greek roots athero meaning "artery," and skleros meaning 'hardening" or "scarring." Atherosclerosis is responsible for the majority of heart attacks, strokes, blindness, and dementia. Atherosclerosis (& inflammation) can be delayed, often by decades. As preventive lifestyles become more common, so will centenarians.

Too many physicians still see plaque-laden arteries as a part the "normal aging" process. A study which is now decades old proved that notion to be false. The China study looked at 50,000 Chinese field workers all the way up to 80 years of age. These workers had no plaque or inflammation. This landmark study should have proved beyond any reasonable doubt that atherosclerosis is not age dependent (although there is a strong correlation in the US), but lifestyle dependent. In other words – what affects the amount of inflammation in our arteries, and the amount of plaque which leads to plaque rupture and ultimately to heart attacks or strokes . . . is what we eat, how active we are, our level of stress, and other lifestyle related factors. (Campbell & TM., 2004) There is little debate that atherosclerosis is the great killer and disabler in the modern, industrialized world. The question is what causes it?

Physicians set out to answer that question over 100 years ago. One of the first hints that the cheesy substance in our blood vessels was a fatty lipid called cholesterol came in 1910. The German chemist Adolf Windaus found that plaques from plaque-laden human aortas contained 25 times the amount of cholesterol as normal aortas. (Goldstein et al 2016). Since then, most of us have assumed what appears to be obvious, that higher concentrations of cholesterol in our blood causes plaque. Over the past few decades, however, interesting questions have come up.

We thought for almost 100 years that the problem was cholesterol in our diet. This has been proven wrong. Why do we still think its cholesterol levels in our blood that cause CV disease? Could that be wrong as well? Cholesterol levels do seem to make a difference, but not as much as previously believed. For example, half the people that experience a heart attack have normal cholesterol values. Doesn't that indicate something else may be as big or even a larger issue?

The debate continues. Some new research has even indicated that higher cholesterol levels are in some cases protective. Why would HDL (often known as "good cholesterol") be so different from LDL (often called "bad cholesterol"). In fact, there is significant debate about the true relative meaning of "good" and "bad" cholesterol.

We think there is gross under-recognition of the role of prediabetes. There is clearly a significant under-diagnosis of prediabetes. Both high blood sugar and high insulin levels have been shown to cause arterial inflammation and plaque. If we are asking questions, what is the relationship between plaque and CV inflammation? It has been demonstrated that plaque formation is driven mostly by CV inflammation. CV inflammation is often driven by high blood sugar and its partner: high insulin values. We share details and definitions of CV inflammation, what causes it, and how to measure it in this book.

So far, we have introduced the problem created by an over-reliance on stress tests for the assessment of heart attack risk. We have demonstrated an example of the human suffering resulting from this over-reliance on stress tests. We also introduced the opportunity to measure CV inflammation and plaque to improve risk assessment. We provide detail behind the biological processes leading to CV inflammation and plaque formation. We also describe a practical way of testing for CV inflammation. The next section of the book details direct inflammation and plaque measurement tests – some which are highly effective . . . and others, not so much.

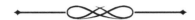

THE TESTS FOR ATHEROSCLEROTIC PLAQUE AND CVD DISEASE

THE FRAMINGHAM RISK ESTIMATOR – NOT A MEASUREMENT, NOT A SCREEN, BUT A GUESS (AND NOT A GOOD GUESS, EITHER)!

Definition

The Framingham Risk Calculator is a predictive equation developed from the Framingham Heart Study. In the early 1950's the US government began a large population study to look at different variables thought to be related to heart disease. This study was renewed and has now spanned many decades of data. The information from this research was carefully studied and analyzed using the most sophisticated biostatistics. These statistics provided an estimator tool based on each individual's comparison to that group of patients, who were followed for decades. The ACC/AHA prevention standards committee recommends that physicians use this risk calculator as a 'first step' in CV risk evaluation. Most initial CV risk assessments now include an estimate of risk based on the use of the Framingham equation.

This estimator begins with medical history and demographics such as age, gender, race. Other risk factors, such as smoking history, are included as well. Each version of the Framingham risk calculator uses slightly different combinations of risk factors. Each set of risk factors result in a score. The various scores are added together for a total risk calculation. The total score translates into 10-year hazard risk ratio or your estimated risk of experiencing an event in the next 10 years.

Framingham is also called the CV Risk Calculator, Framingham Risk Score, and the Framingham Risk App. You can quickly find multiple apps which calculate your risk online. A Google search for "Framingham Risk Calculator" yields 2.4MM hits in 0.5 seconds.

While these risk factors are not unimportant, the over dependence on the scoring tool and the corresponding lack of understanding regarding its inherent weaknesses are leading to missed diagnosis, missed opportunities for treatment, and a continuation of the morbidity and mortality statistics which currently describe this disease. Not too many people would disagree with the premise that any disease, which is nearly 100% preventable (by nearly all accounts), and which still manages to be responsible for a full 1/3 of the deaths in the US, is in an unacceptable state. Worse yet, the trend lines have not moved appreciably in the past 30 years. We must do better!

SUSAN'S FRAMINGHAM/STATIN STORY

Susan is 62 years old. She was taking a 20 mg daily dose of Lipitor (a statin class of drug). She had no evidence of plaque on her CIMT or Coronary Calcium Scores. Her primary care doctor put her on Lipitor because of her LDL cholesterol levels. She asked the doctor about her family history with Familial Hypercholesterolemia (FH) and he wrote the script. He also said something about her CV risk and her LDL levels. Her LDL level was 105. After an informed discussion about the details of the Framingham risk calculator and LDL levels, she decided to stop her Lipitor and monitor her risks until she developed evidence of plaque. Susan's story is not at all unusual.

BACKGROUND

Every CV risk evaluation starts with an estimate, not a measurement. The primary tool is called a risk estimator - the Framingham Risk Calculator. Informed researchers are now calling Framingham a poor guess rather than a calculator. (Kolata, 2013) (Perez, 2016). The current Framingham estimation is often double the actual risk of a patient, leading to unnecessary statin prescriptions. (Cook, 2014). Susan is one such example.

HISTORY OF THE FRAMINGHAM HEART STUDY

Framingham is a small town about 23 miles south of Boston. It is also the home of the largest and most influential cardiovascular risk database in the world. It now includes three separate generations and six cohorts.

What is a cohort? According to Merriam-Webster, the word "cohort" came into the English language in the mid-1500s, along with other terms describing Roman history. (Merriam-Webster, 2019). A Roman cohort was a group of military men that stayed together and shared training and campaign experiences. Over time, the word cohort evolved to refer to any group with shared experiences. In epidemiology (the study of diseases within populations), cohort studies follow groups of study subjects that share an experience or health-related characteristic. The cohort study chronicles the disease process in that group or cohort.

In 1948, Congress commissioned a study of heart disease. The idea was to select and follow a cohort and to see whether lifestyle had an impact on the rate of heart disease development. At that time, heart disease and plaque were considered normal parts of aging. Unfortunately, they still are.

Framingham was chosen over its last remaining competitor, Paintsville, KY. The Framingham Heart Study faced difficulties requiring a management team reorganization during the first year. The situation improved after Dr. Thomas Royle Dawber was appointed the director and chief epidemiologist of the study. Dawber was then chair of the Department of Preventive Medicine at Boston University.

Congress originally commissioned the study for 20 years. At the end of the study, the scientific community wanted to close the study as planned, but thankfully, Congress ignored the scientists' advice and kept it open. At this point (2020), Congress has funded six cohorts and three separate generations of patients. The first was the Original Cohort, founded in 1948. The most recent is the Omni Two Cohort, founded in 2003. Congress' decision to ignore the scientific advisors and keep the study open was a good one. The Framingham cohort has provided over 1,000 published studies. Framingham is the source of the term "risk factor." It is also the most significant source of data for understanding the risk factors for heart disease. For two decades, the Framingham Risk Calculator has been the standard of cardiovascular risk factor estimation.

IS THE FRAMINGHAM RISK CALCULATOR RELIABLE?

The risk estimator emerging from Framingham has its problems. Overuse, misinterpretation, and especially shortcuts have led to unintended consequences. Also, for most of these studies, the Framingham population consisted of predominantly white, Anglo-Saxon men and women. This population is no longer representative of the US population. One study showed that among Japanese American and Hispanic Men and Native American women, for example, the FRS systematically overestimated risk. (D'Agostino, 2001). The most recent (2013) Framingham calculator often doubles the risk calculation, especially in women. (Rospleszcz, 2019).

According to critiques published in The New York Times, such miscalculation led to treatment recommendations (like statins) in far more people than necessary. These conclusions were not just the opinions of medical journalists. These conclusions were demonstrated in studies by well-known researchers, like Paul Ridker and Steve Nissen. (Kolata, 2013) (Cook, 2014).

So why not revert to previous guidelines until the 2013 guidelines can be improved? Because the flawed 2013 guidelines are far better than those they replaced.

Here's an overview of the 2013 Framingham Risk Calculator:

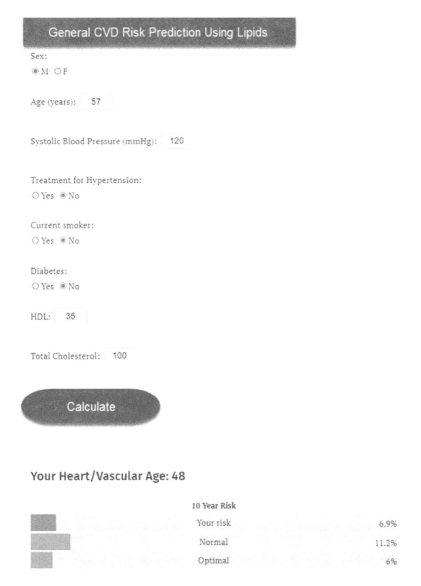

https://www.framinghamheartstudy.org/fhs-risk-functions/cardiovascular-disease-10-year-risk/

Here's another CV risk calculator by UpToDate:

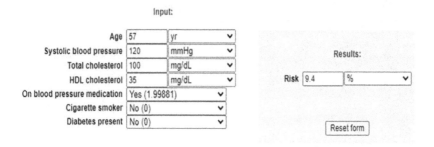

*https://www.uptodate.com/contents/calculator-cardiovascular-risk-assessment-
10-year-men-patient-education*

The Framingham Risk Calculator influences many people to go on statins. Medical standards recommend starting the process with an app, so the physician is instructed to download the Framingham Risk Calculator. The standards committees advise the physician to initiate a patient consultation by entering the patient's key risk factors (like age, cholesterol levels, smoking history, etc) into the calculator. The physician then bases lifestyle and treatment recommendations on the calculator's risk estimates.

WHY ARE THE ESTIMATES SO FAR OFF?

There are several problems with the calculator. First, it assumes a linear and equal relationship between each of the risk factors. What this means is that the model assumes that changes within a risk factor all have the same impact on disease. For example: "The model suggests that lowering systolic blood pressure from 130 to 100 is nearly as important as from 180 to 150," says Dr. H. Gilbert Welch, a professor at Dartmouth. "I doubt there is a cardiologist in the country that believes that." Roger Blumenthal and Micheal Blaha of Johns Hopkins pointed out that the calculations could be improved by including "nontraditional" risk factors, such as CRP (C-reactive protein) or coronary calcium scans. (Kolata, 2013).

As Ford can tell you from his experience supervising thousands of doctors in preventive practices, there are other problems. For example, few doctors go through the entire risk calculation. Doctors are humans; they often shortcut the process. This shortcut is usually something simple such as picking a simple LDL number (like 100 or 130) and they recommend statins based on the subsequent score. But even when followed in meticulous detail, Framingham still causes problems. (Cook, 2014) (Kolata, 2013)

IMPROVING THE FRAMINGHAM RISK CALCULATOR

As described earlier, CV inflammation drives heart attack risk. There are other options for CV testing which could enhance true assessment of CV risk. Wouldn't the inclusion of those "nontraditional risk factors" improve the Framingham Risk Score? That has been the point of a continuing debate. More than once, the US Preventive Services Task Force (USPSTF) assessed the addition of "nontraditional" risk factors.

In its 2009 review, the U.S. Preventative Services Task Force (USPSTF) included "nontraditional risk factors." The term "nontraditional risk factors" included many tests and several technical terms. We list them here because this book is about this debate. Included in this list of 'non-traditional' risk factors were hsCRP (high-sensitivity CRP), ABI (Ankle Brachial Index), Leukocyte count, Fasting Blood Glucose level, Periodontal Disease, Carotid IMT, Coronary Calcium Score, Homocysteine Level, and Lp(a). In its 2018 review, the Task Force found that the addition of these "nontraditional risk factors" improved the risk calculations significantly. (USPSTF, 2018)

Yet, the USPSTF did not recommend any changes to the Framingham risk calculator. Why? According to the committee, there was no evidence that the improvements from using these new technologies would actually help physicians or patients make better choices. "The USPSTF concludes that the current evidence is insufficient to assess the balance of benefits and harms of using the ABI, hsCRP level, or CAC score in risk assessment for CVD in asymptomatic adults to prevent CVD events" (USPSTF, 2018)

We have a different opinion, and we are not alone. We agree with Dr's Blumenthal, Blaha, Cook, Ridker, Naghavi and a host of others suggesting inclusion of nontraditional risk factors would significantly enhance risk prediction capabilities and accuracy. Progress is slowly moving toward this goal. This book includes a section which describes a few of the challenges inherent in all medical standards committees.

Several things are certain: The science continues to develop, these standards committees continue to meet, and the medical standards continue to improve, or at least change their recommendations. One other thing is certain: Preventable heart attacks will continue to occur while this change process takes shape. This book is written for those who wish to avoid those preventable heart attacks. Unfortunately, patients must spend too much time learning this information if they are to significantly improve their chance of avoiding a CV event. It is a small price to pay for enhancing what could be additional decades of healthy and disease-free living.

STRESS TESTS – A LOUSY WAY TO MEASURE PLAQUE.

DEFINITION

A stress test is a procedure used to measure how the heart works during physical activity. These typically involve assessment of heart function while exercising on a treadmill, exercise bike, or drug-induced heart stress. Stress tests are by far the most common method of looking for cardiovascular risk and disease. Stress tests demonstrate high rates of false-positive and false-negative tests, primarily when used to predict heart attacks and strokes. Even conservative medical standards bodies like the American College of Cardiology, the American Board of Internal Medicine Foundation, and the American College of Family Practitioners agree that stress testing is over-utilized for heart attack prediction.

Other names and types of these stress tests include Stress EKG, Exercise EKG, Exercise Electrocardiogram, and Functional Testing (as opposed to anatomical imaging) of the coronary arteries. There are multiple types of stress testing: Nuclear, Echo, and Drug-Induced Stress Testing. These have various names, such as Stress Echo, Nuclear Stress, and Drug-Induced Stress Test. By far, the most common stress tests are the nuclear stress tests. Over eight million of these tests are performed every year. Even within the nuclear stress testing category, there are specific sub-categories, such as SPECT and PET scans.

LONNIE'S STRESS TEST STORY

"I was born in New York. I am 41 now. About 15 years ago, I was playing basketball and had these funny feelings in my chest. I went to the ER. Soon after that, I was getting a stress test. I have had them every year since then. I do not know what they're trying to find.

"It's ok with me, though. Because I still worry about these flutters in my chest. I have had them with annual treadmill tests and cardiology consults. I also had a few Holter monitor tests. They tell me I have Paroxysmal Supraventricular Contractions. They say they are like off-track beats. They also say that I am fine. These things occasionally happen in young, healthy men that work out a lot."

Lonnie is a 41-year-old man in great shape. He does not need an annual stress test. The radiation exposure of having this test repeated every year starting from age 41 significantly increases his lifetime risk of cancer. This compares to a relatively low risk of heart attack or stroke pursuant to his well-understood condition.

MARY GRACE'S STRESS TEST STORY

"My cardiologist recently said the only thing they could see was a slight abnormality in my heart – not anything serious. I had a nuclear stress test a year ago, and now he recommends another. Is this necessary? I read nuclear stress tests should not be given every year, so I feel like I should cancel it. I have also had an electrocardiogram and I have another echocardiogram coming up." – Mary Grace, 63, Florida (Gluckman 2019)

This is another example of a misuse of the nuclear stress test. The 'slight abnormality' needs to be defined in terms of future risk (prognosis) and treatment. What are they hoping to find with these additional tests? More abnormalities? If they find them, what is her prognosis and what treatment (if any) is indicated?

BACKGROUND

The concept behind stress testing is a simple one. It is, however, the fatal flaw in all the stress tests. If there is plaque impeding flow in the arteries which supply blood to the muscle of the heart, stressing the heart will exacerbate the problem, and the condition will be clearly visualized in the test. The first question is the following: which stress test results specifically indicate an abnormal decrease in blood supply? The answer to that question is complicated and it is not very reassuring. The problems continue to come from this key design flaw.

The indicators of ischemia (decreased blood supply) are not that clear. There are multiple categories of indicators. First, there are symptoms, like breathlessness, nausea, dizziness, and numerous types of chest pain. Doctors terminate stress tests early when they see any of these problems. Most stress tests which are terminated early are considered positive for CV disease or vascular obstruction. There are also numerous categories of indicators of ischemia, depending on the type of stress test. For example, EKG or cardiogram stress tests can show problems with the shape of the EKG curve (wave form) or rhythm. Other types of stress tests (e.g., nuclear) show image abnormalities such as an enlarged heart chamber, or a leaky heart valve.

FLOW STUDIES

SCREENING METHODS & "FLOW" STUDIES

It is unfortunate that stress tests are the most common methods for "detecting plaque" today. The misinformation created from the assumption that stress tests predict heart attacks is responsible for countless deaths every day.

The phrase "detecting plaque" is in quotes for the following reason: stress tests DO NOT measure plaque. Stress tests are assumed to elicit signs of decreased blood flow. Stress tests are "flow studies," a term we introduced earlier. The assumption here is that blood flow is inversely proportional to plaque size or the size of an obstruction. Blood flow compromise (as indicated by a hemodynamic disturbance) is not detected at all in stress tests until there is at least $\geq 50\%$ occlusion (blockage) of the artery. Most heart attacks (over 2/3) occur with less than 50% blockage. (Falk 1995).

You can better understand the principle of hemodynamic disturbance and its relationship to blockage by turning on your garden hose. Test how far you need to kink your hose before you affect a change to the flow out the end of the hose. If you notice carefully, you see only minor changes when half of the hose is kinked. If you kink the end of your hose 70% or more, the water will spray out the end as if you had a sprinkler head attached. The spray occurs because you are pushing the same amount of water (the volume) thru a smaller sized hole. This creates pressure and increases the velocity of the water as it comes out the end of the hose. The principles of hemodynamic change affect the velocity and flow of virtually any liquid.

What a flow study measures are changes in velocity. When a velocity increases to a pressure which is indicative of a hemodynamic disturbance, it can be clearly visualized and measured in wave form, or color doppler, or virtually any of the technologies mentioned above. It is important to understand, however, that the only thing these technologies are measuring is this change in velocity. None of these technologies tells you whether there is atherosclerotic inflammation or plaque developing in the arterial walls – they only tell you once that disease process has escalated far enough to cause a blockage which is severe enough to be measured (e.g. $\geq$ 50% blockage).

Many of us know someone that had a negative stress test. How can they be sure they have no plaque in their arteries? Tim Russert, Davie Jones, Gary Shandling, and Alex Trebek all fell into this category (68% of heart attack victims that had less than 50% occlusion or blockage of the artery prior to their actual event) (Falk 1995). Each of these individuals was pronounced 'negative' or in other words they were told they had no blockage. Despite their 'clean' stress tests, each of them went on to have a heart attack.

Routine ultrasound examination of the carotid arteries in the neck does not help either, for all of the same reasons that stress tests don't work in any but the most seriously obstructed patients (e.g. blood flow vs. plaque measurement). The difference between CIMT and the usual carotid ultrasound (e.g. Carotid Duplex) is an additional computerized analysis and measurement of the exact amount of inflammation and plaque (when present) as visualized in the thickness of the intima-media wall of the artery. That is why it is called a CIMT (Carotid Intima-Media Thickness) test. The CIMT test doesn't look at the amount of blood flow or the velocity of that blood flow. It look directly at the artery wall and measures, in millimeters, the amount of inflammation (thickness) or plaque inside the arterial wall. For most people who experience a heart attack or stroke – they had no blockage of blood flow or increase velocity until minutes before their event. What they DID have was plaque and (in most cases) arterial inflammation which could have been there for decades.

PREDICTION OF HEART ATTACKS

For reasons already stated, stress tests do not predict heart attacks well. Most heart attacks occur in people without enough plaque to impede flow. This is true of the majority of patients (68%) who have a heart attack or stroke until minutes before they have one. A full one third of the 'positive' stress test results (e.g. those who are told they have an obstruction which warrants a surgical intervention) are subsequently classified as false positives. (Qamruddin, 2016)

This is why medical standards committees have been recommending that doctors and patients direct efforts and resources away from stress tests.

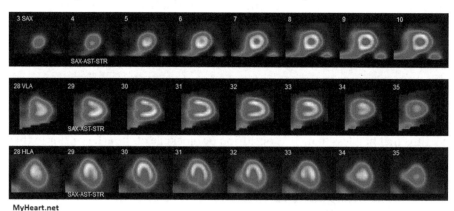

MyHeart.net

https://myheart.net/articles/nuclear-stress-test/

FOUR TYPES OF STRESS TESTS

There are four basic types of stress tests: Stress EKG (or ECG), Stress Echo, Nuclear Stress Tests, and Drug-Induced Stress Tests. There are also other variations of imaging, such as the use of MRI technology (cardiovascular magnetic resonance imaging) or SPECT and PET scanning. SPECT (Single Photon Emission Computed Tomography – and PET (Positron Emission

Tomography) are nuclear imaging tests that use radioactive substances and a special camera to create 3-D pictures). PET (Positron Emission Tomography), SPECT and PET scan stress tests are often together called MPI (Myocardial Perfusion Imaging). Perfusion refers to the passage of blood or fluid (usually a radioactive dye or a chemical) through the blood vessels, usually due to an injection.

DRUG-INDUCED STRESS TESTS

Drug-induced stress tests use drugs to stress the heart and cause the arteries to dilate. A drug-induced stress test bypasses exercise and causes the vessels of the heart muscle to dilate by directly infusing adenosine. While exercising, the body generates energy, using a molecule called ATP (adenosine triphosphate). Adenosine creates dilation of the arteries of the heart and increased pump function. By infusing the body with Adenosine, the heart's reaction to stress can be measured even if the patient is unable to walk, run, or cycle.

STRESS EKG/STRESS ECG

Stress EKG (or stress ECG) is the original stress test. EKG is an acronym for the German word for electrocardiogram. EKG is an electronic cardiac response measurement tool. It measures the electrical pulse or wave forms created via the sympathetic nervous system during complete cardiac cycles. In this test, the patient walks for about 10 minutes on a treadmill. The full process will take about an hour, which includes the time to undress, dress, shower, and preparation time. The doctor creates four records of each stress test. The first is the amount of work as measured by speed and incline on the treadmill. The second is the EKG waveform patterns created during the cardiac cycle. The third is the patient's biometrics (like heart rate and blood pressure). The fourth are any symptoms reported by the patient (i.e. breathlessness, levels of fatigue, or pain).

STRESS ECHO

The stress echo is the same as the stress EKG, except that it adds a cardiac ultrasound or 'echo' before and after the stress events. An operational goal of this test is to get the second echo reading within one minute of the patient getting off the treadmill. Again, the total patient time required for this exam is about an hour, including time to prep and time to undress and dress. The doctor generates the same four records as in the stress EKG. But a fifth is added - the echo or ultrasound reading in response to cardiac stress. The sonographer records doppler images and wave forms which indicate the velocity and direction of flow in each of the chambers of the heart and the vessels leading to and from the heart. It records the size and shape of these vessels and chambers. The live doppler records video of the blood flow in these vessels and chambers throughout the cardiac cycle which provide insight as to whether there is blockage or other anomalies, and how much blockage … provided, of course, that it exceeds 50% or more.

NUCLEAR STRESS TEST

The term 'Nuclear' refers to the use of a small amount of radioactive materials to better visualize the area of interest. In the mid-90s, just over half of all stress tests performed (59%) included nuclear imaging. By 2009, the percentage had swollen to 87%. (Ladapo, 2014). Over 8 million nuclear stress tests are now done each year in the US. This test is similar to the stress EKG and stress echo. Instead of adding an EKG or cardiac echo, this test adds radioactive thallium tracers which are injected into the patient. It takes about 15 minutes to give an intravenous infusion of this tracer, and it can take a couple of hours to read the distribution of the tracer.

The typical patient involved time for a nuclear stress test is 3 to 4 hours. In the nuclear version of a stress test, the doctor supplements the four records (work, symptoms, biometrics, and EKG) with images of the radioactive thallium tracer as it pulsates through the patient's vasculature.

SPECT & PET STRESS TESTS

These two tests are subcategories of Nuclear Stress Tests. SPECT (Single Photon Emission Computerized Tomography) uses a radioactive tracer to generate images tending to be more detailed than other nuclear imaging tests. PET (Positron Emission Tomography) uses a radioactive tracer to create images more precise than other stress tests. PET and SPECT stress tests are considered a subcategory of stress tests called MPI (Myocardial Perfusion Imaging).

CRITERIA FOR ENDING A STRESS TEST

At the beginning of the BACKGROUND section above, we mentioned that there are a lot of clinically prudent reasons to terminate a Stress Test. Below is a list of criteria for ending a stress test early. Early termination of a stress test usually leads to a trip to the catheter lab.

TABLE 1. INDICATIONS FOR TERMINATING EXERCISE TESTING

- Absolute indications
- A decrease in systolic blood pressure of 10 mg Hg from baseline despite an increase in workload, when accompanied by other evidence of ischemia
- Moderate to severe angina
- Increasing nervous system symptoms; (dizziness, or near syncope)
- Signs of poor perfusion (cyanosis or pallor)
- Technical difficulties in monitoring ECG or systolic blood pressure
- Subject's desire to stop
- Sustained ventricular tachycardia
- ST-elevation (another type of EKG change)

Relative indications
- ST or QRS changes (still other types of EKG changes)
- Arrhythmias (more EKG changes)

- Fatigue, shortness of breath, wheezing, leg cramps
- Bundle branch block (more EKG changes)
- Increasing chest pain
- Hypertensive response

(Gibbons, 1997)

CORONARY ANGIOGRAPHY – A DEFINITIVE TEST. INVASIVE, EXPENSIVE, PAINFUL & OFTEN LEADS TO STENT PLACEMENT

DEFINITION

The coronary angiogram is a procedure that uses X-ray to form images of the coronary arteries by injecting a radiology dye into the veins. The injection is usually done using a catheter inserted into the femoral artery at the groin and threaded up through the aorta to the heart. Other names include Coronary Artery Angiogram, Catheter Angiogram, Heart Catheterization, and Cardiac Catheterization.

ALEX'S CARDIAC CATH STORY

Six years ago, Alex scheduled an appointment with a cardiologist at his wife's insistence. He failed a stress test and underwent a cardiac catheterization. The results showed he had a blockage, but the doctor said it was not severe enough to treat.

Recently, Alex scheduled another visit. His wife also prodded this visit. He had shortness of breath and fatigue. Although the cardiologist was different, the results were the same. Alex failed the stress test and had another cardiac catheterization. This time, the cardiologist told him he needed triple bypass surgery.

Put off by the "scary details" and the "pushy" nature of a cardiovascular surgeon who recommended surgery immediately, Alex opted for a second opinion. Through online research, he found Dr. Michael Cortelli, chief of adult cardiac surgery at Memorial Cardiac and Vascular Institute and made an appointment.

Dr. Cortelli was not convinced that Alex needed surgery and suggested a visit with Dr. Juan Pastor-Cervantes. Dr. Pastor-Cervantes is an interventional cardiologist. He is also the medical director of the cardiac catheterization laboratory at Memorial Cardiac and Vascular Institute.

Dr. Pastor-Cervantes scheduled another cardiac catheterization, this time in Memorial's high-tech catheterization lab. The procedure determined that only one vessel required treatment. Alex went to Memorial Cardiac and Vascular Institute's robotic angioplasty suite – the only facility of its kind in Broward County – where Dr. Pastor-Cervantes used a robot for the precise placement of a stent.

"We were able to do the entire procedure through his wrist, and Alex was up and walking within two hours," Dr. Pastor-Cervantes said. In comparison, Dr. Pastor-Cervantes noted that surgery would have involved a large, mid-sternal incision, invasive procedures, a hospital stay of five to seven days, and an extended recovery period.

"When it's needed, it's needed," said Dr. Pastor-Cervantes. "But in this particular case, Alex needed to have just one, only one stent. And that's what we did."

This story does not define what the doctor meant by "it's needed." It appears to be an advertorial for "Memorial's high-tech catheterization lab."

Unfortunately for the hospital, this story does not provide the reassurance that the hospital intended. What this story does demonstrate is the frequent lack of agreement between physicians about treatment plan recommendations following a study that is assumed by many to be the 'definitive test' - a coronary angiogram. If coronary angiograms were definitive, why aren't the recommendations coming out of them just as definitive? This story came from the web site of Memorial Healthcare System in Hollywood, Florida. https://www.mhs.net/news/2015/09/cardiac-cath-patient-story

BACKGROUND

Coronary angiography is not a test for screening healthy people of any age. It is not as dangerous as it may sound, but it still involves injecting a needle into the femoral artery in the groin and threading a catheter tube through the aorta to the heart.

HOW ARE CORONARY ANGIOGRAMS PERFORMED

The area is cleaned and shaved. The doctor injects a local anesthetic and then punctures the skin and the femoral artery with a large needle. A catheter is threaded through the skin and into the artery using a dilator/guidewire combination. The doctor watches an Xray video screen to guide the catheter's progress through the aorta to the heart. The patient usually does not feel anything in the chest but does feel pressure in the groin.

The catheter design allows the use of various tips for specific tasks. Examples include measuring blood pressure in the heart chambers, viewing the interior of the blood vessels, taking blood samples, or removing a tissue sample from inside the heart. The doctor injects dye into the arteries of the heart and takes a set of rapid Xray images. These demonstrate the filling characteristics of the coronary arteries.

Following the procedure, the patient must lie with a pressure bandage at the area of the catheter's insertion for several hours to avoid excess bleeding of the femoral artery. Bleeding remains the most common complication following invasive angiography.

Cardiologists often include further consent or even bypass graft agreement in the consent forms for an angiograph. The stent or bypass grafts are then possible while the patient is in the angiograph procedure using a single sedation. As you can imagine, catheter lab consent forms can be tricky. (Curzen, 2005)

HISTORY OF THE ANGIOGRAM

The first angiogram was completed in 1927 by Portuguese physician Egas Moniz at the University of Lisbon. It was an angiogram of the vessels of the brain. The first heart catheterization was done in 1929 by Berman physician Werner Forssmann. First he inserted a tube in the cubital vein of his arm. Then, he guided the tube up to the right chamber of his heart. He took an X-ray to prove his success. His work was then published on Nov 5, 1929, with the title Die Sondierung des Rechten Herzens (translation: "The Probing of the Right Heart"). (Meyer, 1990).

Dr. Mason Sones, a pediatric cardiologist at the Cleveland Clinic, did the first coronary arteriogram in 1958. (Loop, 1987). It was an accident. He was imaging the aorta, which was not a particularly unusual procedure. As he guided the catheter to the origin of the aorta, injected the dye, and took an X-ray, however, he got a picture of an artery supplying the muscle of the heart, instead of the aorta.

The patient's heart stopped beating for 6 seconds. He was able to restart the heart by having the still conscious patient cough, and the patient's heart rhythm returned to normal and demonstrated no permanent damage. Many of us would have been frustrated with missing the aorta and stopping the heart, but Dr. Sones was excited about the newfound possibility of coronary angiography. After seeing images of coronary angiograms, it is easy to understand why he was so excited. This discovery had the promise of opening a whole new area of medicine. In fact, it did.

Look at the images on pages 73-75 (below) of the arteries coming from an angiogram.

https://youtu.be/N3a2bBnfJO8

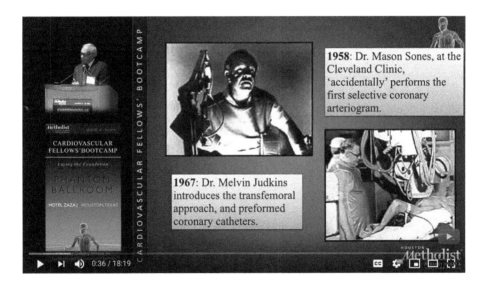

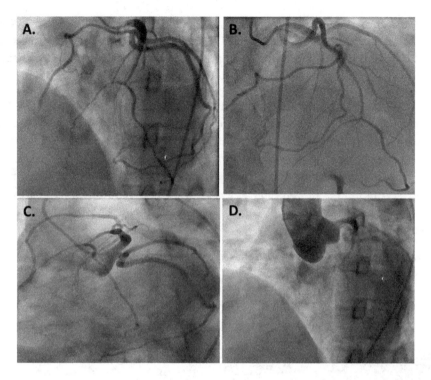

Source: Heart -Coronary Angiogram-ref-heartjnl-2019-July-105-13-998-F1

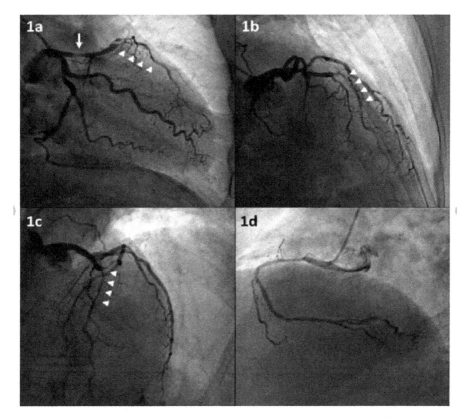

Diagnostic coronary angiography. (a) Left coronary artery, right caudal (spider) projection; (b) Left coronary artery, right cranial projection; (c) Left coronary artery, left cranial projection; (d) Right coronary artery. Severe proximal stenosis (long arrow) and subocclusive mid and distal large stenosis (arrowheads) in left anterior descending artery ((a), (b) and (c)). Diffuse disease in right coronary artery (d).

Source: Heart -Coronary Angiogram-ref-heartjnl-2019-July-105-13-998

Why are coronary angiograms prescribed? The top reasons currently listed for performing a coronary angiogram are measurement or evaluation of:

- Angina, chest pain, or other pain suspicious of coronary artery disease
- Suspicious findings of a stress test
- The function of the right and left sides of the heart
- The capacity of the left ventricle (the workhorse of the heart)
- Cardiac dysrhythmias
- Valvular heart disease

- Myocardial (heart muscle)diseases
- Congenital heart diseases
- Heart failure

The first two reasons above are, by far, the most common reasons for prescribing an angiogram. Multiple medical practice standards committees have stated that coronary angiograms are used too often, especially in conjunction with those first two reasons.

PROCEDURE RISKS

In the early 60s, cardiac catheterization would take several hours, and involved significant complications in 2-3% of the patients. Today, the procedure takes only 1-2 hours, and complication rates have improved to less than 1%. Death occurs at a rate of less than 0.05% or 5 in 10,000 (Manda, 2018)

It is important to understand that between 1 and 2 angiograms per 100 still result in a significant problem. The most common issue is bleeding from the femoral artery in the groin at the injection site. Occasionally the guidewire tears an arterial wall. The femoral artery is a large, high-pressure artery. Of course, the procedure can disrupt unstable plaques poised for rupture, it can also dislodge blood clots. There is always a risk of infection. Also, the process is uncomfortable, time-consuming, and expensive.

Although there is a national cardiac cath/stent registry, there is no routine summary report of deaths from catheter angiography. (Moussa, 2013). Because of this, we must estimate death rates using existing reports. Mortality rates have ranged from .05% to .25% (or between 5 and 25 per 10,000). Multiplication of those rates by the millions of US cath lab angiographies leads us to conclude there are approximately 800 - 2500 deaths annually from angiography. Not all these deaths should be credited to the procedures alone. This is because catheter lab deaths are much higher among individuals with known serious disease. In other words, many of the patients that die had serious known CV risk before the catheter lab angiography. Still, coronary angiograms carry risk.

Some cardiologists slip into thinking these procedures are risk-free, out of habit. A friend of mine once managed a catheter lab. He walked in late one evening to find one cardiologist placing a catheter in the other one. They took turns 'cathing' each other to see what it was like on the patient side of the procedure. While it is usually a good thing when a doctor walks in their patients' shoes, my friend was concerned about the $20,000 expense. Others would be concerned about the inherent risk of performing an unnecessary procedure, especially when it is an invasive procedure.

The most significant risk in coronary catheterization and angiography is not catheter-related injury, it is the unnecessary stent or bypass and further delays in treatment (e.g. the lifestyle changes that would slow inflammation).

If your cardiologist forgets about the risk of injury during a catheter procedure, you may want to read or hear Cricket's experience:

"They made it sound like it was like the smallest deal ever, so I kind of thought it was going to be like giving blood...and I'd be walking around just a few hours later… I really didn't recover for a full two weeks, so I feel like, you know, I wish I had known that before I had this procedure…"

Source: "Angiogram: What I wish I'd known before the procedure."

https://youtu.be/UFOBt33avpw

NONPROCEDURAL RISKS

As previously mentioned, the most significant risk of this procedure is not procedural but the false sense of security leading to complacency. Consider the COURAGE, ORBITA and ISCHEMIA trials. (Boden 2007) (Al-Lamee 2018) (Herman, 2019). These large clinical trials published on a global stage have all shown that stents and bypass grafts do not prevent heart attacks. Stents and bypass grafts may not even cure angina as we have assumed. Although angiograms may identify a plaque, we need to avoid the logic trap that any plaque needs a stent. The most significant debate now involves the assumption that angina requires a stent.

The ORBITA trial indicates it does not. (Al-Lamee 2018) Doctors and patients assume stents fix the problem. The science suggests they do not. Although it may be counterintuitive, this book addresses the real and underlying mechanism of a heart attack to help readers understand why.

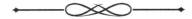

CAROTID INTIMA-MEDIA THICKNESS (CIMT) TESTING

What is IMT and How is it Measured?

As has already been discussed, Intima-Media Thickness (IMT), and the more commonly used term Carotid Intima-Media Thickness (CIMT) is a measurement of the intima and media layers of the carotid arteries using B-mode (brightness mode) ultrasound. In IMT, measurements are taken from the Intima-Media border to the Media-Adventitia border. One or many measurements can be taken depending on the specific protocol which has been prescribed.

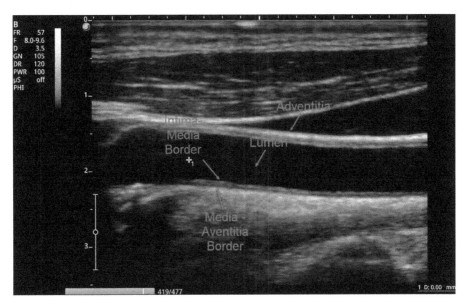

The most useful protocols use a combination of both methods. For example, an average mean is taken from several images of both the right and left carotid or femoral arteries which is used to assess the amount of active inflammation in an individual's arteries at the time of their exam. This is followed by a single or several individual IMT measurements which look at the thickest areas of interest such as plaque. This part of the protocol helps to assess the size and characteristics of any atherosclerotic plaque lesions.

What is Medical Ultrasound and How is it used in IMT?

Ultrasound is a non-invasive technology which means that it does not invade the human body using a scalpel, needle or other invasive cutting tool. In fact, the technique requires no disrobing, it requires no needles, or sticks of any kind, and there is no radiation exposure as a result of the use of sound waves. The exam should be completely painless and can be completed in a manner of minutes.

Sound waves are passing through our bodies all the time. They are harmless. Sound waves pass through us from the radio, from people talking, from electric wires which emit low level sound waves, etc. In short, sound is all around us. However, when we concentrate sound waves through a transducer and we use equipment designed to focus those waves and capture them as they bounce off surface areas, we call this ultrasound.

Generally, the frequency of these sound waves, in terms of their medical imaging potential, is in the range of 2.0 to 18 MHz (Megahertz) (Carovac, 2011). Without overexplaining sound waves, it is important to understand that all sound waves are vibrations which induce waves as they pass through a physical medium. We can measure the amplitude (volume or loudness) of these signals by the height of the sound wave which is measured in decibels (dB). The frequency of these waves is the number of cycles or wavelengths per second or Hertz (Hz). So, when we refer to a megahertz (MHz), each MHz is 1 million Hertz or 1 million wave form cycles per second.

A medical ultrasound exam at 12 MHz, for instance, is one where the frequency of the waves is around 12 million waves per second. These are amazingly fast wave forms which enable us to create pictures, in real time, by bouncing millions of soundwaves off the various mediums in the body (e.g., bones, skin, blood vessels etc.).

In brightness mode (B-mode), the sound waves bounce off dense medium or material such as bone or calcium and send back a signal which appears as a bright white image on the screen. Liquid material, (e.g., blood, water, or puss), bounce back in a dark signal – absent any white pixels or black on the screen. In this manner, trained technicians and physicians can make out bone and muscle structures in a black and white (and shades of grey) structures on their screen – but they can also see right inside of an artery or vein in real time.

Pignoli and the Origins of CIMT

In the early 80's a young, but up and coming researcher and Cardiologist specializing in angiograms in Milan, Italy, was experimenting with ultrasound and human tissue. He and his team discovered a novel use of B-mode (brightness mode) ultrasound demonstrating that the technology could be used to visualize atherosclerotic plaque in a human artery. (Pignoli P. , 1984) Subsequent publications improved the method which launched a landslide of intellectual interest for the potential application of the method on subsequent research and even clinical use. (Pignoli P. T., 1986)

FDA clears for use as Surrogate Endpoint

Carotid IMT has been a widely accepted imaging surrogate marker of generalized atherosclerosis since the late 1990's when landmark epidemiological studies emerged linking IMT to clinical events. (Bartels, 2012), (Chambless, 1997), (Bots, 1997), (O & Leary, 1999). As a result of the correlation between CIMT and clinical events, the FDA began allowing pharmaceutical companies to use the method as a surrogate endpoint.

From a practical standpoint, what this means is that in a large-scale pharmaceutical trial, where drug manufacturers wanted to measure the efficacy of their new drug or therapy and its effect(s) on heart attack and stroke reduction, the FDA would now allow these companies to measure the effect on each patient's CIMT instead of waiting for a certain number of clinical events (e.g. heart attacks and/or strokes) to take place in the control group.

Prior to this change, drug companies had to wait for a representative population sample to have a heart attack or stroke in order to measure the outcomes derived from their drug or therapeutic. This could take years or even decades to track and, now that a less provocative tool had proven effective . . . it was now unethical to allow individuals in a control group to go on and have their heart attack or stroke. The implications are a huge reduction in the costs associated with completing a pharmaceutical trial, and a significant decrease in the amount of time it took to observe measurable results. Lower development costs mean lower cost of these drugs to patients.

Without going into a lot of unnecessary detail to demonstrate this point, suffice it to say that it would be challenging to find a drug currently on the market for the treatment of heart attack and stroke risk factors, which does not have a study on file involving the use of CIMT.

One example appears on the package insert for Rosuvastatin (Brand Name: Crestor), which includes as one of the indicated uses for the drug: "to slow the Progression of Atherosclerosis". This indication (or recommended use) was justified because of a study 'Measuring Effects on Intima Media Thickness: an Evaluation Of Rosuvastatin 40mg' (METEOR). (Crouse, 2007). Another example was in the Arbiter trial where CIMT was used as the primary justification for the release of a new therapeutic: Niacin. (Taylor, 2002).

Once again, you would be hard pressed to find a drug or therapeutic currently on the market for the treatment of heart attacks and/or strokes, or any of the risk factors for the same, which does not have a study on file with the FDA involving CIMT and the effect(s) of that drug or therapeutic on CIMT. This is because the FDA recognizes that CIMT is an early indicator of who will and who will not go on to experience a heart attack and/or stroke.

We have no intention of citing every study the FDA used to justify approval of a cardiovascular therapeutic in this book, but simply want to demonstrate that the modality has been used and continues to be used as a surrogate endpoint for decades – in order to demonstrate that the modality has clearly been accepted to be a "safe, noninvasive, and relatively inexpensive means of assessing subclinical atherosclerosis." - This from the American Heart Association's EXPERT panel on Atherosclerosis. (Greenland, 2000).

Landmark studies document relationship between CIMT and Disease

Over the years, several longer-term studies have been classified as "landmark" because their contribution to the science of atherosclerosis and a better understanding of the pathogenesis and even pathophysiology of heart attacks and strokes, that they have become essential reading to those charged with treating the disease. Let us review a few of those studies.

Perhaps most important as it relates to establishing a relationship between CIMT and both heart attacks and strokes, is the Atherosclerosis Results in Community (ARIC) study. Since 1985, the ARIC community surveillance data has provided unique insight, in a rigorously validated methodology, on the incidence and fatality rate of coronary heart disease in US populations.

The ARIC study consisted of two components: community surveillance and then a study cohort. Study participants were recruited from four economically and racially diverse counties (Forsyth County, North Carolina; Jackson, Mississippi; eight northern suburbs of Minneapolis, Minnesota; and Washington County, Maryland). (https://www.nhlbi.nih.gov/science/atherosclerosis-risk-communities-aric-study).

The ARIC study originally enrolled approximately 16,000 adults who have been monitored for >30 years. The study helped assess rates of heart attack, hospitalizations from heart failure and deaths due to heart disease in > 400,000 adults. This on-going research has led to over 1800 peer-reviewed published articles on heart disease. Because of the significance of the effort, the number of years the study has been on-going, and the amount of new science that is derived from its research . . . the study will forever be considered 'landmark'.

The ARIC study was the first landmark study to establish an association between coronary heart disease and IMT as well as a relationship between stroke and IMT. The ARIC study showed a significant increase to the hazard rate ratio (a person's future risk of heart attack or stroke) for each 0.19mm of increase to IMT. (Chambless, 1997) (Chambless L. F., 2000).

Other landmark studies which showed similar, yet important new relationships between IMT and both cardio (heart attacks) and cerebrovascular (strokes) disease include:

EVA (Etude sur Ie vieillissement arreriel, the Vascular Aging Study) - showed that each increase of 0.10mm in CIMT resulted in an 18% increased risk in future cardiovascular events. (Bonithon-Kopp, 1996)

The Rotterdam study – demonstrated that CIMT had additional value beyond traditional risk factors in cardiovascular risk stratification. A closer look at the data revealed that over 60% of the cohort would have been reclassified to either a lower or higher risk compared to the group they were placed in using traditional risk factors. The Rotterdam study showed the odds ratio (or risk) of stroke increased by 51% for each 0.163mm increase in IMT and this was true in BOTH men and women. (Elias-Smale, 2011) (Iglesias del Sol, 2001);

The EAS (Edinburgh Artery Study – showed that small changes in IMT were associated with clinically significant development of atherosclerosis in the peripheral arteries (Allan, 1997).

The KIHD (Kuopio Ischemic Heart Disease) - demonstrated a relationship between traditional risk factors like LDL and HDL cholesterol levels, CIMT, and atherosclerosis. The study showed that each 0.1mm increase in IMT resulted in an 11% increase in risk of MI. (Salonen, 1988);

The CHS (Cardiovascular Health Study) - another four-community study which looked at factors related to the onset and course of coronary heart disease (heart attack) and stroke. The CHS study found that CIMT was an independent predictor of both heart attacks and strokes – especially when one looked at plaque as a function of CIMT, and not just the average of the mean. This study also showed that risk was elevated for each 0.2mm increase in IMT (Simon, 2010).

Each of these studies, and the thousands of subsequent research papers that were published relating to their initial work, can easily be found using a simple Google Scholar search. The slight differences between risk ratio to IMT measurement has mostly to do with the different protocols that were used in each of these studies.

The important and consistent take away is this: An increase in IMT = increased risk for future heart attack and/or stroke. It is that simple. What is important is not that these studies took place, but that they are each rigorous multi-year efforts which demonstrate an important and independent link between IMT and the disease which is responsible for over 70% of the heart attacks and strokes. To date, there are over 14,000 peer reviewed, published research papers using IMT. That amount of research simply does not occur in technologies that have not been proven effective.

Outcomes: One 10- year 100,000 person-year study that the skeptics cannot ignore

If you wanted to read just one study, who's science was so good that it would compel you to believe that CIMT is perhaps the most important test available to predict your personal risk of a future heart attack and/or stroke and to monitor whether on-going therapy prescribed is working . . . then you should read this section of our book.

In 1990, a group of researchers familiar with the relatively new B-mode IMT technology to evaluate carotid and femoral arteries, struck out to understand whether this technology could be useful in an asymptomatic (no signs or symptoms of disease) and otherwise low-risk population (people like YOU!). (Becaro, 2001)

To identify their cohort (the study population) they looked at a randomly selected population sample of over 14,000 adults. Then, they systematically eliminated from participation all those who had elevated LDL or HDL which was too low. They eliminated from the study all those with elevated blood pressure, anyone with renal or metabolic problems or genetic diseases. Only those patients with blood tests within the normal range were included in the study.

This was important, because they had each participant sign an agreement to NOT receive any treatment for cardiovascular risk factors during the 10-year study – and that would not be ethical in a population with risk factors for disease. To be clear, none of these participants would have qualified for a pharmacological intervention – but it is important to understand the effort that was made to eliminate from the study ANYONE who had any of the traditional risk factors for this disease which were known at the time.

Once the study population was selected, they proceeded to monitor these patients every two years using IMT measurements as the primary monitoring tool. It is important to understand that the researchers used BOTH carotid AND femoral IMT measurements in their study. This is important because as many as 20% additional at-risk patients can be identified by looking at BOTH carotid and femoral IMT.

We must remember that ALL measurements of the intima-media layer INCLUDING plaque is an IMT measurement. However, in research settings and even among some physicians, there is a general mis-understanding that somehow IMT and plaque measurements are different. They are not. Plaque is defined by the size of the IMT measurement and its characterization. There are other operational definitions besides absolute size which help to differentiate plaque from normal thickening . . . but nearly ALL IMT measurement >1.3mm are, indeed, atherosclerotic plaque. In fact, nearly all IMT measurement > 1.0mm are atherosclerotic.

Remember, these are metaphorical pimples inside the wall of the artery. When we measure a plaque's size, we measure the lumen-intima interface to the media-adventitia interface to arrive at the thickest area of interest (see Image on page 79). A plaque lesion is often further defined as a lesion where the wall thickness is ≥ 1.0mm AND where the apex of that lesion is >50% of the average measurement directly proximate (closer to the heart side) and distal (further from the heart) from the lesion. In other words, we look at the areas immediately next to all sides of the lesion and if the apex of the lesion is > 50% higher than the areas directly next to the lesion . . . then the lesion is an atherosclerotic plaque.

This is an important differentiation and underscores why many people, including researchers and clinicians, misinterpret their data. In literature, IMT has often been redefined as either the average of several or the average of hundreds of measurements from the right and left sides (usually from the far wall of the common carotid). We also see research protocols which used the single thickest IMT. These protocols will nearly ALWAYS be more predictive of events because they INCLUDE plaque. Protocols which feature the average mean of a group of measurements in the common carotid may or may not include plaque – but they will be much more reproducible.

An ideal protocol will measure the average mean of the common carotid from the far wall (because the far wall is more accessible and more reproducible). This will provide the most accurate assessment of the amount of inflammation in the wall of the artery. The ideal protocol will ALSO provide an assessment of all plaque lesions (areas of interest measuring >1.3mm at the apex and where the apex is >50% higher than the immediate areas surrounding the lesion) found in an area of interest - usually a 3 – 5 cm portion extending from the distal 1cm of the common carotid and/or common femoral arteries and extending into the internal and external carotid arteries or conversely, deeper into the femoral arteries.

Inflammation is predictive of plaque . . . and loosely correlates with events. The reason there is a weaker correlation between the average mean IMT and heart attack or stroke than there is between plaque and heart attacks and strokes is that the average mean of the common carotid generally or commonly omits plaque lesions.

Plaque is most often found in the bifurcation of the common carotid (an area closer to the brain than the common carotid), and in the internal carotids (an area closer to the brain than the bifurcation). Plaque are predictive of clinical events. Remember that ruptured plaque is responsible for >70% of the heart attacks and/or strokes. So, the more of these 'pimples' that are found within the walls of an artery, and the softer they are (meaning the more echoluscent or filled with puss and necrotic or dead material which can easily rupture into the vessel), the more likely they are to rupture.

The average mean measurements of the common carotid artery are a direct measurement of the amount of inflammation in the arterial wall. Whereas distinctive plaque measurements are a direct measure of atherosclerotic lesions which are very predictive of future events. As we have already pointed out... plaques are predictive of events, but inflammation is predictive of plaque. Thus, inflammation is less predictive of future events than are atherosclerotic plaques.

Back to our story – these researchers were monitoring 10,000 adults in their study population. What resulted was astonishing and important to science. 21% of this low-risk, asymptomatic population went on to have either a heart attack or stroke in the 10-year window of this research. This means that 21% of an untreated population that had zero risk factors (using traditional methods), went on to experience a horrific event anyway.

Here is the takeaway: the piece that your physician and every primary care physician on the planet should understand: IMT successfully identified 98.6% of those who went on to have a heart attack and/or stroke and it did so BEFORE they had their event.

To put that number in perspective – a home pregnancy test in the first trimester catches approximately 97% of the pregnancies. So IMT was more effective than a home pregnancy test at identifying those who would go on to have a heart attack and/or stroke – and it identified them BEFORE they had their event. I am not aware of another technology, and I would challenge all who read this chapter to find a single medical technology that captures 98.6% of ANY condition BEFORE it occurs.

We learn from this study a few more important details. 42.7% of patients who have a small unobstructive plaque (a lesion which was so small it did not cause any blockage, it did not cause any hemodynamic disturbance) will have an event within 10 years if left untreated. Hemodynamic disturbances are caused whenever the pathway of a fluid is restricted. For example, if you put your thumb over the end of a garden hose, or otherwise kink the hose . . . how far do you have to kink the hose before it sprays out the end of the hose or makes that hissing sound we have all learned to recognize when our hose is kinked? That kink or spray is a hemodynamic disturbance which can be measured. 87% of patients who have a large obstructive (causing enough of a blockage to cause a measurable hemodynamic disturbance) will have an event within 10 years if left untreated. (Becaro, 2001)

We must remember, this was not a small study, nor was it a 1- or 2-year study. This study followed 10,000 patients for 10 years. That equates to 100,000 person-years of research. This data simply cannot be ignored by even the most skeptical of skeptics.

What are the ramifications for you and me, our friends and family? It is this: If you want those you love to know whether or not they have risk for a future heart attack and/or stroke – they need to get an IMT exam from a laboratory that has a peer-reviewed and published protocol which demonstrates their ability to perform it reliably. The sooner they get this test, the sooner they can get prescriptive advice from their physician to prevent such an event.

If you are a primary care physician, you may be wondering how this will change what you do or how you practice medicine. To you we would say this: We sincerely hope that even in the absence of corroborating blood tests or ANY other test results, you would treat your patient differently when they provide you with images and empirical evidence on a report which demonstrates they have active atherosclerotic disease.

Treatment effects CIMT AND Disease

One of the primary things skeptics have thrown out against IMT is that even if you treated the disease to the effect of reducing IMT progression, there was no evidence that this would result in fewer events. It certainly represented a GAP in the literature. Outcome studies (which is what these skeptics were asking for) are extremely expensive to complete. Who would pay for such a study?

Luckily, such a study was completed midway thru 2020. This original peer-reviewed article showed the effect of reducing CIMT progression on actual cardiovascular events in >100,000 adults. (Willeit, 2021) What had previously been a key missing link to the entire IMT story is no longer missing data.

What the researchers show is the usefulness of CIMT progression as a surrogate marker for cardiovascular disease risk. Their analysis reveals a statistically significant association between TREATMENT EFFECTS on progression of CIMT and the TREATMENT EFFECTS on cardiovascular disease risk.

In other words – if you treat CVD disease (heart attack and stroke risk factors) and use CIMT to monitor the effects of that treatment . . . what you see is strongly correlated and predictive of future CVD events. If you reduce progression of CIMT . . . you will also reduce cardio and cerebrovascular events. If you fail to reduce progression, you will fail to reduce cardio and cerebrovascular events.

This single piece of information should give you the courage to either treat your patients using CIMT to track efficacy . . . or alternatively, if you are a patient, to insist your primary care physician use CIMT, from a reliable laboratory, as a tool to regularly and systematically monitor the efficacy of their treatment for your risk factors.

Weaknesses of the Method

All medical tests have their weaknesses, and CIMT is no exception. The 3 most difficult challenges relating to the weakness of this modality have to do with

1) Operator dependent image acquisition (or getting to the same place in three-dimensional space every time),

2) Operator dependent image analysis and measurement (measurement of the exact same areas of interest),

3) Quality control /assurance of items #1 & 2 and biostatistical rigor to control for all coefficients of variability.

Operator Dependent Image Acquisition

The most obvious of weaknesses pertaining to this test has to do with the fact that it is an operator dependent test. What this means is that even if one could hypothetically perfect the analysis and measurement of the images, one can only measure the image one receives. The quality of the image, the anatomical location from which the image was taken, and at an even deeper level, the actual physics of ultrasound are all effected by the quality and talent of the person taking those images, combined with the unique anatomical challenges and differences between patients.

The images provided by a sonographer (the medical photographer if you will) are all dependent on the anatomical limitations presented to the technologists.

What this means is that although all humans have commonalities between their anatomy, they also have quite different anatomical features which contribute to the complexity of securing quality ultrasound images.

A way to think about this is to think about thumb prints or eyes. Even though most humans have two eyes which feature an iris, a lens, some pigmentation etc. . . . the combinations of these factors make each person's eyes unique to them. The same can be said of finger and/or thumbprints. So unique are these subtle differences between humans, that biometric scanners are routinely used to identify, with exact precision, the individuality of a human such that it can easily identify and differentiate one person from another.

My own laptop computers have biometric controls using either my eyes, my face, or my fingerprint to identify me and certify, biometrically, that I am the actual person attempting to logon to my computer.

In sonography, these differences can occasionally present challenges for the technologist – some which can be overcome with an experienced and seasoned sonographer – some (such as pathologies which block the ultrasound signal) cannot be overcome with even the most seasoned sonographer. However, at the time of this book's publication, no ultrasound school in the country was providing instruction on an IMT protocol, much less instruction on how to get a reproducible IMT exam.

A challenge attributed to the skill of the sonographer has to do with getting to the same place in three-dimensional space. If I want to be able to compare a patient's prior year scan to the current exam, I need to have images which are taken from precisely the same angle, the same depth, and the same anatomical location as they were in the prior year's exam.

Ultrasound schools provide valuable training to their students on how to get to a particular anatomical location. Little or no instruction is provided to these same technologists about how to get to a particular circumferential location. Let me explain what we mean by the circumferential location.

If we imagined that an artery is a round tube (which it is) with 360 degrees of circumferentiality, and then we imagine that same vessel sits inside of an object (e.g. a human neck) which prevents us from moving the camera (or transducer) completely around that tube so that we are limited as to how much of the tube we can access with our transducer or camera, we begin to understand the depth of the problem.

Add to that the fact that these vessels are rarely straight tubes like a plumbing pipe. They curve and undulate and feature curves remarkably similar to a snake on the ground. The ultrasound probe used to capture images can optimize the image on about 3 inches of linear space on that snake. Imagine now we are attempting to capture an image on a particular 3-inch segment of that snake as it moves in the grass. Each curve of the snake requires a different angulation of the camera in order to optimize the image of the particular segment of that snake we need to capture. Hopefully, this helps to articulate just a few of the challenges involved in acquiring consistent images between the same and different patients.

Without launching into a deep dive on the physics of ultrasound waves, what we need to understand is that the rules of physics dictate how sound waves bounce off a surface area. The more curves there are in an anatomical area of interest, the more difficult it is to acquire an image which can be measured reliably. Once again, ultrasound schools are not currently providing specific training on how and where to take these images. It is different than the more traditional uses of ultrasound and requires specific and formalized training.

Operator Dependent Image Analysis and Measurement

We call the technologists who analyze and measure the images provided by a sonographer a 'Reader' because they analyze and measure the images and provide measurable results to a physician who then interprets those results. Even when two independent readers look at the same set of images, absent a prescribed and clearly defined protocol or definition of where and how to take the measurements, there is an enormous amount of variation between readers.

To illustrate this point, let us share a real-life experience Dr. Eldredge had involving training people to 'read' these images:

I was involved in a training many years ago at a conference where atherosclerosis and its prevention were featured topics. A group of approximately 70 physicians met for this medical conference which took place about a decade ago. A training class was available to physicians who were interested in learning more about CIMT. The class was conducted by an extremely competent and skilled physician who had been involved in some especially important research featuring CIMT. Dr. Allen Taylor, a prominent cardiologist at Georgetown University Hospital and chief author of the Arbiter trials on Niacin which featured CIMT as a surrogate endpoint in those studies, was the instructor.

To better illustrate and underscore this point, it should be pointed out that EACH of the physicians attending this 3-day course received the same instruction. EACH of the attendees used the EXACT same set of images so there was zero variability between images. In real life, the largest variability relates to sonographers and we NEVER have the advantage of working off the exact same set of images. EACH of these attendees, however, used the exact same set of images, they utilized the same software to measure these images and they EACH used the same type of computer equipment with similar chips and memory.

Notwithstanding the enormous efforts to minimize coefficients of variability, the closest that ANY two physicians got during this 3-day course was 0.10mm. That may not sound like a huge difference – and, in fact, it is an extremely small difference . . . about the size of a single strand of hair on the average human head. However, this small amount of variability is 10-times greater than what we allow in our own laboratory performance criteria.

That is right – after a 3-day course, taught by a prominent cardiologist, who was VERY experienced in his own use of CIMT, the closest that any two physician students got to one another was 0.10mm which is 10 X higher variability than we can accept from our own laboratory.

Imagine what the variability would be from readers or sonographers or even laboratories who had not received any specific CIMT training and who have no specific protocol to tell them how and where to take the measurements.

This single problem is the number one reason skeptics cite as their resistance to the utility of the CIMT technology. Let us just say that the skeptics are not wrong to be concerned about this.

In the Atherosclerosis Results in Community (ARIC) study, (Chambless, 1997) the landmark study which first tied CIMT to clinical events for both Heart Attack and Stroke, it is important to note that the net Average CCA Mean CIMT difference between the group of patients who went on to have a heart attack and the group who did NOT have events, was only 0.08mm.

Without going into a larger discussion about biostatistics, standard deviation, and statistical significance, (which is covered at length in Dr. Eldredge's #1 International Best Selling Book "Cardiovascular Wellness Management Success Plan") it should be noted that what this means in practice is that if two technologists cannot get their variability to within a standard deviation of <0.02mm . . . they cannot, with any sense of statistical confidence, . . . even tell you who is and who is not likely to have a future heart attack and/or stroke.

This one fact underscores why skeptics have a hard time accepting or buying into this important technology. If a group of physicians sitting in a 3-day class, measuring the exact same set of images, with the exact same software, on the exact same equipment cannot manage their variability to less than 0.10mm . . . how are we to believe that anyone can?

The good news is that the problem has been solved and documented in peer-reviewed published data which we will discuss later. For right now, it is important for you to wrap your brain around the importance of variability to the method and the difficulty of managing that variability between technologists.

Quality Control /Assurance and Control of ALL Coefficients of Variability

If you accept the premise that it is theoretically possible to control these variables via training, the use of specific tools, or any other means necessary ... then you must also accept the absolute necessity of monitoring those tools and the application of those tools in order to preserve the integrity and consistency of their use.

The minimum requirement to manage these variables are documented and reproducible protocols for both image acquisition, and measurement of the areas of interest. The protocols must clearly outline how and where the images should be acquired as well as how and where they should be measured. The protocols should outline specific anatomical markers from each angle to assure image acquisition compliance between operators. The protocol should outline a consistent and demonstrably reproducible training program. What do we mean by demonstratable?

Absent the rigorous post-training testing of those trained in the method, we can never be certain whether the principles outlined in the protocols can be followed in practice. This is not just a function of testing their knowledge via a multiple-choice questionnaire. A multiple-choice questionnaire can assess knowledge, but not application of knowledge. A multiple-choice questionnaire would be grossly inadequate for this purpose.

In order to know of certainty that the protocols can be reliably reproduced in practice, one must test the skill and application of the knowledge via a performance-based certification. Ideally this certification would be double-blind in order to prevent internal bias and skewing of results. The results would be certified by an independent 3rd party.

When technologists are tested in a double-blind, performance-based certification, which is subsequently verified by an independent 3rd party, a laboratory can be certain that its technicians not only understand and have the knowledge about where and how to take the images, but that they can also APPLY that knowledge in a competent manner. They must demonstrate that they have the skills necessary to APPLY that knowledge reliably in a variety of different patients.

At CardioRisk Laboratories, every technologist undergoes such a certification. The certification uses biostatistics to measure each technologist's variability to themselves looking at EVERY coefficient of variability (different patients, different equipment, different technologist, different readers, etc.).

This means each technologist scans the same patient multiple times. We compare each of those exams to each of their additional exams and we quantify the exact amount of variability they have to themselves. We also have other technologists perform the exam on the same patients, in replicate, so that we can measure each technologist's scans to every other technologist's scans, always including at least one technologist who has already completed and passed their certification (the control). This is done on a double-blinded basis (only computer-generated randomized numbers for identification of both technologists and patients are used – the key is sent for safe keeping to an independent 3rd party).

In peer-reviewed and published data of the CardioRisk technologists, the arithmetic difference between the combination of coefficients of variability (e.g., different sonographers, different readers, and different equipment) was 0.002mm with a standard deviation of 0.02mm. (Riches, 2010).

Testing the application of the principles and protocols taught during training is one aspect of quality. However, these are human being with inherent biases, life challenges, and distractions. If training were enough in any field of expertise, then anyone who had learned to correctly hold and swing a golf club could theoretically compete with Tiger Woods. However, even Tiger Woods goes through phases where he fails to apply the lifetime of training he has received.

Anyone who has ever competed in sports at a high-school or higher level can attest to the value of ongoing coaching. We understand intuitively the value of having someone watch our 'play' and then provide us with unbiased feedback as to how we can improve.

In a life-saving technology such as this, ongoing coaching and use of well-defined quality control and quality assurance metrics are the only way to make sure that all those involved in the process maintain vigilance to the defined protocols and quality procedures.

If patients and physicians want to be able to rely on the life-saving data which can potentially be provided via CIMT scanning, then they must get that data from organizations who not only understand this variability, but who have implemented rigorous processes to maintain the quality and application of a well-defined process. Absent such procedures and knowledge, the skeptics would be absolutely correct in their assessment – the methodology would not be nearly as valuable.

Summary of What To Look for When Getting a CIMT:

As we have already discussed, if you now believe that IMT can accurately and effectively predict future events and that it can be used to monitor efficacy of treatment of CVD risk factors - and you have a basic understanding of both the method's strengths and its weaknesses . . . then you will need a checklist (of sorts) of how to select a CIMT vendor and what to look for.

To summarize what we have listed above . . . below are the minimal technical proficiency criteria you should look for before selecting a CIMT laboratory for your own evaluation, the evaluation of your patients, or especially when contemplating clinical research:

Reproducibility – they must have peer-reviewed published data demonstrating their reproducibility preferably via a double-blind, performance-based certification . . . and certified by an independent 3rd party and the ISCIMU (International Society of Clinical Intima-Media Ultrasonography)

Protocol Matters – Have them detail in written format how and where their measurements are taken and what steps in their protocol will assure that images will be taken from the same depth and angle in year over year evaluations of the same patient. In other words – how will they assure their technologists ALL take pictures of the same lesion – and get to the same place in three-dimensional space? There should also be a written criterion for how and where the images are read or measured as the skill to acquire images is different than the skill to analyze and measure the images.

Training and Certification of Technologists – How and for how long are their technologists trained on the specific CIMT and FIMT protocols? Can they provide detailed information on how they train and certify their technologists – (this should include both Sonographers who acquire the images, and Readers who measure the images?) Their technologists should be certified by an independent 3rd party based on a double-blind, performance-based certification. If possible, the methodology and testing should be certified by the ISCIMU. As of the date of publication of this book, CardioRisk Laboratories is the only CIMT laboratory that meets these criteria.

Ongoing QA / QC – Anytime a test involves the skill level of a human, that test is subject to error owing to the proficiency and attention span of the technologist involved. Because IMT is a test requiring proficiency of a human, constant care must be made to have multiple sets of eyes evaluate EACH set of images to make sure they meet the minimum criteria for quality. Quality Assurance and Control must be applied to every aspect of the reporting process. For example:

The Images: Was the protocol followed? Is the quality of each image sufficient to provide meaningful interfaces to measure? Are the key anatomical interfaces clearly visible in all images? If not, are there written instructions detailing what should be done with invalid images or those which do not meet the quality standards?

The Measurement of Images: Is there consistency in the measurements between Readers? How often are blinded re-reads administered to test the competency and proficiency of each reader?

Patient Anomalies: Are there anatomical anomalies which could impair the quality of the results?

Scientific Expertise: Is there a scientific expert or doctor with specific imaging training available at the laboratory to validate and verify that anatomy has not inadvertently been identified as pathology (and versa visa) and to sort out ultrasonic artifact from both pathology and anatomical structures?

If these minimal quality standards are not practiced on each image set, the laboratory performing the tests is at significant risk at reporting erroneous information to those requesting the data.

Hopefully, this chapter has provided you with useful information to help better understand this important technology. More importantly, we hope it has provided you a useful tool to incorporate it into your own life whether you are a provider or a patient. One thing should now be clear, this technology has the potential to extend both the quantity and the quality of human life. This is the one test that can prevent you, your loved ones, and your patients from ever having to experience an atherosclerotic caused heart attack and/or stroke.

JUDI'S STORY

Judi was 68. Her doctor wanted to put her on statins for her age and an LDL cholesterol value of 168. He had calculated her Framingham risk score, which suggested she had a 6.4% probability of an event within ten years if not treated. She had seen too many negative comments about statins on the internet, so she did not want to take them. Judi had been watching several informative YouTube channels on the subject. She focused on Ivor Cummins' and Ford Brewer's channels. She saw the movie WIDOWMAKER. She also had a Coronary Calcium Score of 0. She elected to work on lifestyle changes instead of taking a statin. Most importantly, she focused on weight loss.

Even the National Lipid Association agreed with her. They used her story on their web site, promoting the Coronary Calcium Score and MESA score. Her calculated Framingham Risk score dropped from 6.4% to 2.6% with the zero Coronary Calcium Score. (Goldberg, 2019).

A subsequent CIMT exam revealed what we already suspected: that she had no plaque in either her carotid or femoral arteries. By looking at her other risk factors and then visually inspecting the vessels in three separate vascular beds (Coronary via a Coronary Calcium Score, Carotids via a CIMT, and Femoral via a FIMT exam) we can be more comfortable allowing Judi to continue her path of not taking a statin. Having said that, we have continued to monitor Judi to make sure that her arteries do not suddenly flare up with massive amounts of inflammation, which would indicate she was ripe to grow plaque.

The CIMT exam allows us to continue to monitor Judi's arteries and allow her to stay off her statin until such time as we see an effect of the elevated cholesterol inside her arterial wall. This illustrates how and why a CIMT can be used to bridge the gap found between the standard of care in most primary care offices, and the care received from a Cardiologist . . . which necessarily delays treatment until it is too late. Sometimes this bridge informs us we need to step up the treatment to get more aggressive. Other times, as in Judi's case, it confirms that we can feel confident not treating aggressively for now, while allowing us to keep a close eye on her in subsequent year over year examinations. Armed with appropriate monitoring tools, we have been able to save patients the inconvenience and cost of beginning an aggressive pharmaceutical management program for (in some cases) decades and to do so with absolute confidence that nothing was being missed.

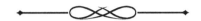

CORONARY ARTERY CALCIUM SCORE

DEFINITION

The Coronary Artery Calcium Score is a measurement of the quantity of calcium in the arteries of the heart using CT imaging. The presence of any calcium, as indicated by ANY Coronary Artery Calcium Score > 0, indicates there is plaque, or atherosclerosis, in the coronary arteries. This test is easily accessible, relatively inexpensive, and well standardized. It is a good screening tool for CV disease. It is NOT great for tracking or monitoring progression of disease. The Agatson Score is a standardized scoring system used to calculate a Coronary Calcium Score. The Coronary Artery Calcium Score is also known as the Calcium Score, CAC, or CACS.

BACKGROUND

The 2018 ACC/AHA Cholesterol Guideline recommends CAC. Their level (IIb) recommendation states the following. "Coronary artery calcium (CAC) testing may be considered in adults 40-75 years of age without diabetes mellitus and with LDL-C levels ≥70 mg/dl-189 mg/dl at a 10-year atherosclerotic cardiovascular disease (ASCVD) risk of ≥7.5% to <20% (i.e., intermediate-risk group) if a decision about statin therapy is uncertain." (Grundy, 2018)

AGATSTON VS MESA

The Coronary Calcium Score starts as an image. In order to compare points in time, individuals and populations, a score is needed. There are several scoring methodologies. The most dominant traditional score is the Agatston score which was developed in 1990. It is a straightforward calculation of the total amount of calcium across multiple coronary artery beds.

The Multi-Ethnic Study of Atherosclerosis (MESA) calculator is new. (https://www.mesa-nhlbi.org/calcium/input.aspx). The MESA calculator incorporates the CAC score in addition to the traditional risk factors of demographics, cholesterol, systolic blood pressure, diabetes, smoking, family history of CHD, and the use of hypertension or cholesterol medications.

The MESA study gave rise to the score calculator. The MESA study confirmed the utility of CAC testing in 2009. (Budoff, 2009). Two years later, the EISNER trial demonstrated a reduction in overall CV risk, without the added cost, using calcium testing. (Rozanski, 2011). Other science supports these findings. The 2013 American College of Cardiology/American Heart Association guidelines gave CAC testing a class IIb recommendation.

It is import to have some understanding of these class ratings. Generally, a class I recommendation indicates it is standard practice and highly recommended. Failure to implement a class I recommendation is equivalent to malpractice. A class II indicates a recommendation which is prudent in some instances. A class III finding is a recommendation to NOT use a technology.

Within each class there are subtypes. A subtype of 'a' indicates there is strong support in the research literature supporting this recommendation class. The subtype 'b' indicates there is moderate support, but some conflicting research and more information is needed. The subtype 'c' indicates there is very weak support in the literature for the technology.

THE AGATSTON SCORE

The Agatston and other traditional Coronary Calcium Score methods have many populations indexed to them. However, they also include incorrect assumptions about the calcification process. This testing and scoring method do not account for calcium in all vascular beds and it uses outdated technology.

This has implications for the definition of a negative score. For example, this technology misses the fact that uncalcified plaque is more dangerous than calcified plaque because it is more vulnerable to rupture and/or erosion. Scientists are evaluating newer methods to mitigate that weak spot. (Blaha, 2017)

HOW CORONARY CALCIUM SCORE IMAGES WORK

Calcium shows up as a bright white area in the image of the coronary arteries. The reader calculates the amount of bright white shown in the picture. The calcified surface areas are then calculated and added together and expressed as a Coronary Calcium Score. The higher the score, the more calcium on the patient's images. The higher the score, the higher the patient's risk of a future heart attack. Coronary Calcium Scores are simple, quick, easy, relatively inexpensive, and painless. Stress tests are not.

Due to the significant radiation from the calcium scan, it is not recommended for young, healthy people. Older equipment can deliver up to 2000 times a single chest X-ray of radiation, whereas some of the newer machines use closer to 10 times the emission of a single X-ray. As more modern equipment becomes available, the radiation doses necessary to secure a quality image will most likely continue to shrink.

NEAL'S STORY

"Doc, I know I've got maybe 6 or 7 years to live. I want to get some things done before I die." Neal was 57.

"Why do you say you've only got 6 or 7 years to live?"

"Because I've got calcium in my heart. I've got a score of almost 300."

The doctor told Neal he should reconsider. By the time men are 57, over 70% have a positive Coronary Calcium Score. 300 is not an excellent score for a 57-year-old, but it is not a death sentence. Neal was over-reacting. As Agatston said, you must find the root cause and change it. Neal was 5 feet, 10 inches, and weighed 240 pounds. He had work to do. If he were successful, he could expect decades more of a healthy life.

The Agatston score has five categories, ranging from 0 to over 400. As you can see in the image below (Image on page 104), a score of 300 is considered a moderate risk.

It is not unusual to see men in their mid-60s with scores over 1,000. With proper risk factor management, these men can expect to make it to their 90s.

In Neal's case, one of our goals was to help him to gain confidence that his Coronary Calcium Score was not a death sentence. He could live for decades more with appropriate management of his condition.

One of the first things we did with Neal was to order a Carotid Intima-Media Thickness (CIMT) exam – not because we were necessarily looking for plaque – we know Neal has plaque . . . but because we wanted to track the active disease in the wall of his arteries as reflected in the amount of inflammation found in his arterial wall. On Neal's initial exam, we were alarmed not just at the amount of plaque in his carotid arteries, but also the amount of active disease reflected by the inflammation in his carotids. Neal was only 57 when we met him, but his arteries were the equivalent of someone >80 years of age.

This enabled us to get aggressive with Neal's treatment. A course of action was prescribed first involving diet and exercise. This was followed by the implementation of a statin, some blood pressure and diabetes medicine. Neal had metabolic syndrome which is why he was gaining belly fat.

Today we can celebrate the fact that Neal has lost 40 pounds. He is off his diabetes and blood pressure medications. He continues to take his Statin because of the plaque in his arteries – but amazingly, the inflammation in his arteries has steadily declined in year over year CIMT exams.

In Neal's last exam, his arteries were equivalent to a 50-year-old male, which is much younger than Neal's 61 years of age. The plaque in Neal's carotids have progressively stabilized from being on the softer side of heterogenous to being mostly calcified. This means that Neal's long-term risk of a future event has been significantly attenuated. More importantly, he has stopped worrying so much about whether or not he will make it thru the end of the year.

Neal continues to exercise regularly and reports a new zest for life. The psychological aspects of health improvement cannot be understated. Imagine the comfort of believing that instead of having months or a few years to live

. . . you could live decades longer. Such is the value of appropriate disease management when combined with regular testing and at least annual monitoring.

We have known how to treat this disease for over 50 years. The gap in health care has to do mostly with the fact that we continue to significantly **under-diagnose.** Nobody needs to have an atherosclerotic heart attack or stroke, much less die from one.

Table 3 · **Calcium Score Distribution (Calcium Score – Agatston Score) and Confidence Interval**

Percentil	Sample values	[95% conf. interval	MESA study values*
5	0	0 – 0	0
10	0	0 – 1	0
25	10.5	1 – 55.1	0
50	176	78.9 – 360.7	13
75	626	446.6 – 856.8	97
90	1757.4	859.3 – 2712.8	303
95	2699	1743.9 – 6114.9	555

Percentiles estimated for white, 57-year-old asymptomatic males, with previous coronary or vascular disease, in the MESA study (The Multi-Ethnic Study of Atherosclerosis).

Source: https://ctscanmachines.blogspot.com/2018/05/ct-scan-calcium-score-range.html

CCS (Agaston)	Risk	Description
0	Non-identified	Negative test. Findings are consistent with a low risk of having a cardiovascular event in the next 5 years.
1-10	Minimal	Minimal atherosclerosis is present. Findings are consistent with a low risk of having a cardiovascular event in the next 5 years.
11-100	Mild	Mild coronary atherosclerosis is present. There is likely mild or minimal coronary stenosis. A mild risk of having CAD exists.
101-400	Moderate	Moderate calcium is detected in the coronary arteries and confirms the presence of atherosclerotic plaque. A moderate risk of having a cardiovascular event exists.
>400	High	A high calcium score may be consistent with significant risk of having a cardiovascular event within the next 5 years

Source: https://ctscanmachines.blogspot.com/2018/05/ct-scan-calcium-score-range.html

RADIATION AND THE CORONARY CALCIUM SCORE

We cover the risks associated with all the CV imaging studies later in this book. The radiation picture with Coronary Calcium Score is unique among those studies. The test is not harmless, but the radiation danger is minimal compared to CV risk in middle-aged individuals. The Coronary Calcium Score uses CT, and therefore Xray. It is not entirely harmless as it exposes the patient to radiation. Because of the radiologic exposure, there are no screening studies of young, healthy people like there are with CIMT.

CALCIUM AND SOFT VS CALCIFIED PLAQUE

Plaque goes through cycles of worsening and improving. As plaque heals, it becomes fibrous and calcified. Calcified plaque is safer than soft plaque by factors higher than 6x. (Honda 2004). This fact creates a paradox: If calcification is a sign of plaque healing and stabilization, then why are higher Coronary

Calcium Scores indicative of greater risk? There is some evidence that higher Coronary Calcium Scores represent higher overall plaque generation. But this topic is, in fact, one of the challenges of the traditional Coronary Calcium Scores like Agatston.

Does this mean that patients with a relatively low Coronary Artery Calcium Score could still have soft plaque, even though there is no calcium? The simple answer is 'YES'. The Coronary Calcium Score does not detect new or soft plaque. A couple of times each year, we see patients who have deceptively low Coronary Calcium Scores who have soft plaque as imaged in a CIMT exam. One of the viewers of Ford's YouTube channel, Lisa Rector, described this experience in her husband's arteries (see Image below).

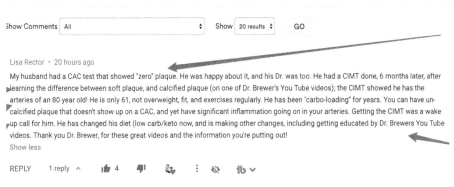

Source: Ford Brewer YouTube Channel

LISA RECTOR: COMMENTS ON DR. BREWER'S YOUTUBE CHANNEL:

"My husband had a CAC test that showed 'zero' plaque. He was happy about it, and his Dr. was too. He had a CIMT done 6 months later, after learning the difference between soft plaque and calcified plaque (on one of Dr. Brewer's YouTube videos), the CIMT showed he has the arteries of an 80-year-old. He is only 61, not overweight, fit, and exercises regularly. He has been 'carbo-loading' for years. You can have uncalcified plaque that does not show up on a CAC, and yet have significant inflammation going on in your arteries. Getting the CIMT was a wakeup call for him. He has changed his diet (low car/keto now and is making other changes including getting educated by Dr.

Brewer's You Tube videos. Thank you, Dr. Brewer, for these great videos and the information you're putting out!"

Is that true? Is Soft Plaque More Dangerous than Calcified Plaque? The answer is 'YES'!

FRANK'S STORY

"But doc, you don't understand. If I have got any plaque at all, I want it gone. I want to get rid of it."

Frank was 63, with an arterial age of 69 (IMT of .82 mm), and 3 discrete plaques greater than 1.3mm.

He discussed the following with his doc. A complete reversal of plaque is not a practical goal. Plaque is much more likely to be reversible if it is less than three years old, and sometime this is the result of a ruptured or eroded arterial wall, not an actual regression of the plaque.

Calcified plaque tends to be more difficult if not impossible to get rid of. Calcified plaque is usually filled with connective (scar) tissue and collagen as well as calcium and other minerals. It is older in the disease process, but stable. Frank's history indicated his plaque deposition occurred more than three years earlier, probably due to smoking and obesity. Frank's CIMT, showed that his plaques were calcified.

"Well, if you tell me that I can never do any better, I guess I'll have to accept that."

SOFT PLAQUE VS. CALCIFIED PLAQUE

A study by Dr. Osama Honda and associates, published in 2004 demonstrated that calcified plaque, as measured by carotid intima media thickness (CIMT) testing is stable. The study "Echolucent carotid plaques predict future coronary events in patients with coronary artery disease" was conducted in Japan by Dr. Osama Honda. (Honda, 2004) The images from the paper should jump right out at you.

Low-IBS Plaque

High-IBS Plaque

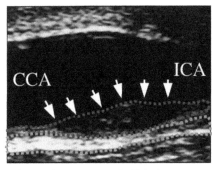
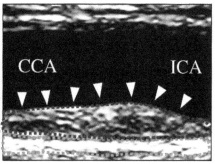

Plaque (intima-media)-IBS: 34.6	Plaque (intima-media)-IBS: 44.7
Adventia-IBS: 52.2	Adventia-IBS: 52.2
Calibrated-IBS: -17.6	Calibrated-IBS: -9.1
IMT: 2.1	IMT: 2.3

Source: (Honda, 2004)

As you can see, the image on the left shows "low IBS plaque." This is also called "soft" plaque, "hot" plaque, or in this study, "echolucent" plaque. The image on the right shows "high IBS plaque," also referred to as calcified or "echogenic" plaque. "Echolucent" lets ultrasonic waves pass through without any echo; "echogenic" plaques reflect the ultrasound waves.

These differences are not just subjective visual impressions. The following optical measurements were taken to make them objective (a measurable number).

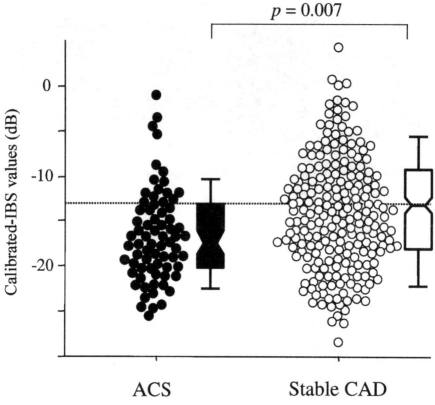

Source: (Honda, 2004)

The authors then followed these patients for an average of 14 months (up to 30 months) for CV events. Of 112 patients with soft plaque, 29 had events. Of the 103 patients with calcified plaque, only 4 had events. This happened even though the calcified plaque was slightly larger in size than were the soft plaques. In other words, the size of the plaque was significantly less important to future events than was the presence or absence of calcium.

Table 3
Summary of Coronary Events During the Follow-Up Period in Patients With Stable Coronary Artery Disease

	Echolucent Carotid Plaque		
	With (n = 112)	Without (n = 103)	p Values
Total coronary events	29	4	< 0.001
Cardiac death	4	0	
ACS	19	2	
Non-fatal acute myocardial infarction	2	1	
Unstable angina	17	1	
ACS treated with			
PCI	11	2	
CABG	3	0	
Medical alone	5	0	
Recurrent angina (sudden hospitalization)	6	2	
Invasive therapy	4	2	
Medical alone	2	0	

ACS = acute coronary syndromes; CABG = coronary artery bypass graft surgery; PCI = percutaneous coronary intervention.

Source: (Honda, 2004)

The average IMT of the calcified (echogenic) plaque is 2.3. The average IMT of the soft (echolucent) plaque on the left is 2.1. Think about the risk for these individuals. For patients with soft plaque (29 out of 112 patients): (29 patients/112 patients) x (14 months/12 months) x 100 = 30%. Compared to patients with calcified plaque (4 patients/103 patients) x (14 months/12 months) x 100 = 4.5%

These were notable differences between the two patient groups and a nearly 7-fold increase in event risk.

BONUS TAKE AWAY:

You may be wondering about what this means and why this information is important. While we will not spend too much time on this, it is important to note that one of the most important attributes of the statin class of drugs is that they have been shown to attract minerals like calcium and collagen to the wall of the plaque. This is important.

Calcium and collagen indicate that these lesions have stabilized. This means the risk of heart attack and stroke is greatly reduced. Unfortunately, this important drug attribute is nearly lost on all but the most discriminating physicians and patients. Marketing has effectively labeled these drugs as 'cholesterol lowering' drugs. They certainly do that. However, a more important feature of the Statin drugs may lie in their ability to reduce inflammation in the arterial wall, repair the endothelium lining, and attract minerals such as calcium and collagen to stabilize plaque lesions.

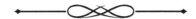

THE CT ANGIOGRAM –LOTS OF POTENTIAL, BUT NEEDS TO BE STANDARDIZED IN TERMS OF RADIATION AND USE

DEFINITION

The CTA (Computerized Tomography Angiogram) is a measurement of plaque and the anatomy of the coronary arteries using intravenous X-Ray dye and CT imaging. Recent studies indicate this could add additional clarity to the standard stress testing. There has been a rapid "learning curve," resulting in the need to encourage the use of the CTA and the use of the latest equipment to avoid radiation.

"Much data in support of the diagnostic accuracy and prognostic value of noninvasive coronary angiography by computed tomography have emerged within the last few years. These data challenge the role of stress testing as the initial imaging modality in patients with suspected coronary artery disease." (Arbab-Zadeh, 2012)

ARNOLD'S STORY

"Doc, I can't believe you're saying the same thing as those other docs," Arnold looked at his doctor (Ford) with disappointment. "I thought you were different. You are the 4th doctor to tell me, 'I can't find a problem. But you need to take a statin.'"

Ford acknowledged he was the 4th doctor to recommend a statin, but unlike the other doctors, he had found a significant problem - plaque. You just needed to know where and how to look.

Arnold was 63 when we first met him. He had been out fishing with his 14-year- old son and fainted. In the Emergency Department, the doc worked him up in detail for potential stroke or heart attack. He told us the doc said, 'I really can't find anything wrong. But you should probably start taking this statin,' and handed him a prescription for atorvastatin (Lipitor).

Arnold did not like the idea of taking statins. He also did not like not knowing what caused the symptoms. He went to an internist who said, "I don't know what happened. I can't find anything wrong, but I recommend you take this statin." He went to a cardiologist who put him through a stress test. He passed it. The cardiologist, in turn, had no recommendations other than statins.

Then Arnold came to see Dr. Brewer. Arnold's CIMT test was normal, with an arterial age of 58 and no discrete plaque. We told him that that between 2 and 4% of CIMT tests could be false negatives. Occasionally plaque develops in the arteries of the heart but not the carotids. While it is highly unusual, it does happen in less than 5% of patients. We cover a couple of these examples in this book.

Arnold asked about the possibility of a false negative result on a stress test. False-negative stress tests are much more frequent, so we advised him to ignore the stress test.

Arnold had an elevated CRP. All patients seeking a CV risk assessment should have an OGTT (Oral Glucose Tolerance Test) with insulin values.

Arnold did have a significantly elevated CRP, so we suspected early insulin resistance. His blood sugar challenge with an OGTT (a more definitive test for prediabetes - see the glossary) was borderline. Still, his A1c was 5.7 which is within the recommended reference range (A1c - or HgbA1c is a blood test that looks at average levels of blood sugar over an approximate three-month period. It helps detect diabetes and prediabetes). See glossary. The normal range is < 5.7, so this is right on the border of prediabetes. Arnold's basal insulin was 7 (the normal range is usually <5 mIU/L . A value of seven indicates prediabetes). Insulin response to the glucose challenge was not available at the time.

Arnold also had an LDL of 98 (current recommendations would indicate that this should be <100 for people with no known health issues, but lower if they are diabetic or pre-diabetic). To the credit of all previous doctors, that is at least a standard approach recommendation for a statin. But Arnold declined the LDL approach for statins.

We discussed getting a Coronary Calcium Score, and we mentioned a CT angiogram (CTA). He was getting more frustrated with the lack of explanation for his fainting episode.

He asked for the more definitive CTA. We considered a Coronary Calcium Score first, especially since the findings were so subtle. However, Arnold was continuing to accumulate a lot of costs over the workup for that fainting spell and it was clear he was going to continue to dig at this—he was already discussing a nuclear stress test.

So, we ordered the CTA. We found that he had a plaque in the Left Anterior Descending (LAD). Regionalized disease (in the area of the heart but not the carotids or other vascular beds) is more common in people with congenital heart defects or in people who have had surgical work on their heart.

According to the report, it was "not occlusive." I explained to Arnold that he had a plaque and that it did not need to be occlusive to cause a heart attack. It just needed to be soft and then subsequently rupture or erode, releasing its content into the bloodstream to form a clot. Some CTAs will give indicators of plaque stability (calcified versus soft). Arnold's CTA indicated the plaque was calcified.

Arnold's case indicated early-stage and erratic blood sugar problems. We do not recommend statins for LDL values (except in rare cases of the genetic disease familial hypercholesterolemia). Statins are recommended whenever there is documented atherosclerosis as evidenced by his plaque. The fact that plaque was present indicated that Arnold had been through cycles of insulin resistance and even inflammation.

Upon hearing the recommendation for low dose rosuvastatin (generic Crestor), Arnold made the comment about four doctors recommending statins despite no findings. Again, plaque in the LAD, the "widowmaker" artery of his heart, was not a "no findings." Like most of us, Arnold was emotional about the discovery of plaque in his arteries. Most of us go through some denial when we first find a plaque in our arteries. He did overcome that initial denial, took the medication, and made necessary changes in his lifestyle.

Many physicians are familiar with patients whose worry about their condition exceeds what the best science tells us about their disease. Frank's concerns related mostly to the few fainting spells he had experienced, which he had subsequently decided were related to cardiovascular disease and impending doom.

The small amount of plaque in Arnold's lower descending artery finally convinced him to begin a low-dose statin. The statins would stabilize any disease he had in his entire vasculature, repair any damage to his endothelial lining, and arrest any existing or future inflammation in the walls of his arteries. Part of the challenge with Arnold was in managing his worry. By explaining the disease process to him thoroughly, and subsidizing that explanation with annual test results, we were able to calm his concerns regarding any future events.

Four years later, Arnold's CIMT results continue to show he has healthy arteries. At Arnold's insistence, a subsequent Coronary Calcium Score was completed which showed a slightly higher amount of calcium. Because Arnold now has a better understanding of his disease, he knows this is a good result, not a negative one. There is nothing approaching a blockage, so the increase in calcium is related to more stable plaque that poses very little danger of a future rupture or erosion. The fact that this plaque is now stable significantly lowers his future risk of CV events. Arnold is still anxious – but has increased his exercise regimen to daily largely due to feeling confident that the fainting spells were not related to some future CV event.

BACKGROUND

CT angiogram is also called CT angiography or CTA. It is typically performed in a radiology department or an outpatient imaging center. The technology uses X-ray with catheters, CT (computerized tomography) or MRI (magnetic resonance imaging), and contrast material.

CTA is a minimally invasive test. It typically combines an injection of iodine-containing contrast material and CT scanning to examine the arteries supplying blood to the heart and to determine whether there is a plaque in these arteries. The images generated during the CT scan are reformatted to create three-dimensional (3D) images that may be viewed on a monitor or film. We typically receive written reports along with a CD containing the images.

The CT scanner is typically a large, box-like machine with a hole or tunnel in the center. The patient lies on a narrow table that slides in and out of the box. The machine includes a ring called a gantry. X-ray tubes and detectors appear on opposite sides of the ring. The gantry rotates around the patient. There is a computer workstation with a technologist nearby who speaks with the patient throughout the exam.

The big difference between a coronary CT and other CT scans is the speed of the CT scanner and the use of a heart monitor. The unique challenge of coronary CTA is scanning the arteries. This challenge stems from the fact that blood vessels may move 5 or 6 times the distances of their radius with each beat of the heart (Budoff M. , 2006)

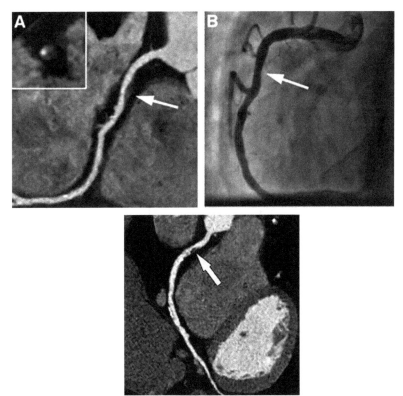

Source: https://imaging.onlinejacc.org/content/4/11/1227/F1

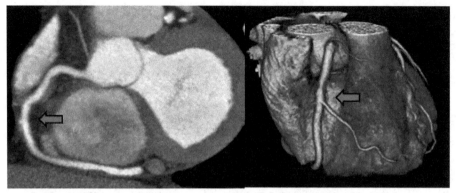

*Source: https://www.londoncardiovascularclinic.co.uk/cardiology-info/
investigation/ct-coronary-angiography*

TWO LANDMARK STUDIES OF CTA

THE PROMISE TRIAL

The PROMISE trial was the first big study showing the potential for CTA to bolster the current stress test problems. The final sentence of the first publication reads as follows. "Coronary CTA, by identifying patients at risk because of nonobstructive CAD, provides better prognostic information than functional testing in contemporary patients who have stable chest pain with a low burden of obstructive CAD, myocardial ischemia, and events." (Hoffmann, 2017).

PROMISE was a multicenter trial. Patients with stable chest pain were randomized to get either a CTA or "functional testing" (e.g., exercise EKG, nuclear stress, or stress echocardiography). It is essential to differentiate the functional testing described in this study from the functional testing we describe elsewhere in this book. The type of functional testing described in this study have also been described in this book, but they are significantly different from those described in the section on Vascular Function Testing.

In this study, patients were followed for 26.1 months. The endpoints were death, myocardial infarction (heart attack), or unstable angina hospitalizations. The ability of CTA to predict such events was significantly better than that of the functional testing group described in this study.

The PROMISE trial was a "non-inferiority" trial. What does "non-inferiority" mean? It is a term that medical researchers use to show that the test or treatment studied is "at least as good as" something else, usually the standard of care test or procedure. Researchers randomized the angina patients to the stress test of the doctor's choice. The term 'functional' is used because they include assessment of vascular function following some form of exercise. There are three common types of functional stress tests: Stress EKG, Stress Echo, and Nuclear Stress Tests. We have already discussed all of these tests earlier in this book.

The PROMISE trial showed that CTA performed at least as well as any of these three stress tests at managing patients with angina.

As stated by the last sentence of the PROMISE study, you could make a case that CTA is better than the other technologies. Of course, more evidence is needed. That is just what the SCOT-HEART Trial provided, and which is described next. This trend to demonstrate significant advantage of CTA over the various types of stress tests appears poised to continue.

THE SCOT-HEART TRIAL

The SCOT-HEART Trial is a vital step in the science concerning CTA. In this trial, one group or cohort received the "standard" evaluation while the other group had the "standard" plus CTA administered. "Standard" refers to whichever of the 3 'standard' stress tests the physician wanted to do at the time of the clinical workup. (The SCOT-HEART investigators, 2015).

CTA found increased numbers and severity of lesions, which led to increased treatment and long-term improved outcomes. However, care should be used in interpreting that last statement. Most would assume that "increased treatment" means "increased stenting". That is not the case. In fact, those who received the "CTA + Standard" testing got more treatment via all types of invasive procedures (e.g., stents, bypasses, AND preventive treatments) during the first year. But these treatments were less frequent in years 2 to 5, and the patients in the test group lived longer.

Overall, the SCOT-HEART Trial made a strong statement in favor of CTA. What happened in this trial? The patients that had the CTA saw actual images demonstrating their increased risk for heart attack and stroke. They were far more likely to make life-saving changes in their habits. We see this phenomenon often when someone realizes they have a plaque using less expensive and less invasive techniques like Coronary Calcium Score or CIMT. The image of a plaque in your arteries, especially plaque which is a mere 3 or 4 inches from your brain, creates increased motivation to adhere more strictly to the prescribed intervention. This allows the patient to drop those carbs, lose those pounds, get off the couch, develop proper sleep hygiene, and other habits that will extend their lives. This is especially true when patients can monitor their progress as they can with CIMT.

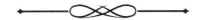

VASCULAR FUNCTION TESTS

DEFINITION

Vascular Function Testing is a group of non-invasive tests which measure the abilities of arteries to expand (dilate) and constrict in response to challenges. These tests can be helpful but require advanced quality systems to be reliable.

BACKGROUND

As we have already described in this book, the arterial wall has 3 layers: the intima (which includes the endothelium and the structure directly beneath this one-cell thick layer), the media, and the adventitia. Each of these layers has individual roles in the circulatory system. The intima regulates vascular tone, permeability, and the metabolic exchange of cellular nutrients and wastes. The media is the primary determinant of elasticity, which regulates continuous delivery of blood to the tissues. Failure of these functions results in damage to the artery walls and tissues supplied by the arteries. Several non-invasive methods are currently used to assess vascular dysfunction. (Tomiyama & Yamashina, 2010).

The most popular tests in this category include Flow-Mediated Dilatation (FMD), Pulse-Wave Velocity (PWV), and the Augmentation Index (AI). Endothelial function is assessed by the FMD and contributes to the progression of atherosclerosis. Increased arterial stiffness is assessed by the PWV and AI. Arterial stiffness contributes to increased blood pressure, impaired coronary blood supply, atherogenesis, and microvascular damage. (Tomiyama & Yamashina, 2010). Other tests include PAT (Peripheral Arterial Tone) and Digital Thermal Rebound (DTM). PAT measures the response to stress in a post-occlusive (following artificial blockage of the artery) measuring amplitude signals from the flow of blood and the changes between pre and post occlusion. DTM uses temperature changes to estimate vascular function. DTM also measures blood flow (via Digital Thermal response) in pre and post occlusion. The idea in both PAT and DTM is to measure a reactive hyperemia (see Glossary). Reactive hyperemia is the transient increase in blood flow which occurs following a brief period of ischemia (lack of oxygen in the vessels) usually due to deliberate and short-term (less than 5 minutes) arterial occlusion (blockage).

For a more complete description of the link between vascular autonomic function, endothelial function, permeability, and stiffness, see the following articles or contact CardioRisk Laboratories 801-855-6775. , (Kawagishi & Matsuyoshi, 1999), (Smulders, 2000), (Stehouwer, 2004), (Stehouwer C. H., 2004), (Stehouwer C. S., 2006)

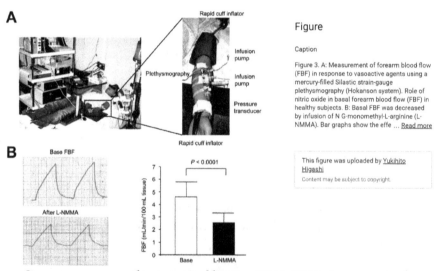

Figure

Caption

Figure 3. A: Measurement of forearm blood flow (FBF) in response to vasoactive agents using a mercury-filled Silastic strain-gauge plethysmography (Hokanson system). Role of nitric oxide in basal forearm blood flow (FBF) in healthy subjects. B: Basal FBF was decreased by infusion of N G-monomethyl-L-arginine (L-NMMA). Bar graphs show the effe ... Read more

Source: www.researchgate.net/publication/273149092_Assessment_of_ Endothelial_Function/figures

VASCULAR FUNCTION TESTING – WHAT THEY MEASURE - AND WHY

Non-invasive vascular function tests can provide additional information to biomarkers and structural testing (like CIMT). They require robust quality control structure and processes outside the scope of most clinics. These tests are usually best obtained as part of a package of services from a high-quality supplier, such as CardioRisk.

The intima lines the entire arterial system, all 60-100 thousand miles (depending on the age of the patient) of it. The endothelium provides crucial metabolic functions such as fuel, oxygen, and waste exchange with the cells. The intima protects the artery walls from oxidized LDL and other pathogens which lead to plaque formation. Lastly, the intima is the source for NO (Nitric Oxide), one of the essential chemicals made to dilate or expand the arteries. When workload expands (like running uphill), more oxygen is required by large muscles such as the heart and the legs. The arteries need to dilate the vessels feeding these muscles to increase blood flow and oxygen supply.

These functions involve multiple mechanisms and structures, ranging from parts of the brain recognizing the biochemical indicators to NO production by the intima to relaxation by muscle cells within the media of the artery wall. During all this, specialized nerve centers (the autonomic nervous system) must function correctly for proper vascular function.

As many now understand, erectile dysfunction is a failure of the vasodilation function in the penis of males. It is also a significant known risk factor for CV disease. Drugs like Viagra and Cialis create a vasodilator function similar to NO where they help to dilate the vessels of the penis so that the blood flow maintains an erection. Unlike NO, however, these drugs are targeted to a specific area of anatomy. In practice, drugs like Cialis and Viagra are now routinely prescribed for other vascular function improvement and are routinely used daily by some patients.

It may be helpful to briefly discuss why this type of testing makes both clinical and statistical sense in terms of screening, diagnosis, and ongoing monitoring of the disease progression/regression.

The largest organ in the body is the endothelium. The endothelium is a one-cell thick lining which lines all 100,000 miles of an adult patient's circulatory system, and every organ in the body. The endothelium performs several important functions in terms of cardiovascular health. First, it is a protective lining which functions very much like a Teflon coating. It protects the inner layers of the artery from perforation by pathogens (disease-causing cells) for 4, 5, and sometimes even 7 decades of life.

Second, the endothelium is the source for nitric oxide, a natural substance which serves as a vasodilator (it makes the arteries expand). This is an essential function of vascular tone, for moving the blood effectively through the vessels and for responding to increased workload on the body's large muscles. After decades of use and abuse, this layer gets compromised and perforated, rendering it less effective. When the endothelium is compromised, natural vascular function is also compromised. This can result in plaque formation, or inelastic arteries that have reduced capacity to respond to necessary environmental changes of the body (e.g. increase workload).

It is not uncommon to see advertisements for erectile dysfunction medication (i.e. Viagra, Cialis). These drugs contain vasodilators which target sexual organs which have been compromised. In the case of erectile dysfunction, however, the physician prescribing drugs never knows if that dysfunction is caused by psychological factors (the patient's mental well-being which can adversely affect this function), a pharmacological factor (some drug the patient is taking can adversely affect this function), or a physiological factor (something inherently wrong in the patient's circulatory or arterial function which adversely affects this function). What is known is that the patient's vessels no longer fill with blood to cause an erection when they should. (Vlachopoulos, 2015).

Erectile Dysfunction is just one example of what can happen when vascular function is compromised. Another way to visualize vascular function is to think about long-distance running or any type of rigorous exercise which is performed for an extended period of time.

If you have ever gone for a rigorous run for more than 15 minutes, you have likely experienced the phenomenon known as "the second wind". This phenomenon is one of the body's most dramatic demonstrations of vascular function.

In a normal and healthy individual who begins to run at a moderate to fast pace, the body sends a series of signals which keep it healthy during and throughout this increase expenditure of energy. Although we have simplified the description of what happens, the essential elements of physiological change have been outlined below:

First, the heart and other large muscles such as those in the legs, send a signal to the brain that they are working harder and are in desperate need of oxygen. The brain then verifies that the heart and other muscles need more air. It then sends a signal to the endothelium and other vessels which feed these muscles (this one-cell thick layer which lines every vessel in the body) to release nitric oxide.

As we have already discussed, nitric oxide is a natural vasodilator which immediately causes the vessels of the heart to expand. This dilation or expansion allows more blood to be carried to and from the heart to other areas of the body. The blood, of course, carries oxygen – so that all of the essential muscles, appendages and organs of the body that were previously under stress due to the increased workload, are now able to receive their increased oxygen and return to a state of homeostasis or equilibrium.

Although this process is carried out using the body's autonomic neural system, many regular exercisers will attest to the fact that they can sense or feel their body's response to this process. It is a phenomenon know as "the second wind".

Note: some functions such as breathing we cannot mentally cause to stop or start. The body takes care of these functions without our conscious input. These processes are part of what we call the 'autonomic neural system' because we can't 'will ourselves' to stop breathing or to stop doing other life-essential functions performed by our body – our body self-protects these functions by taking them out of the control of our conscious mind).

This phenomenon of getting our vessels oxygen is often referred to as "a second wind". This phenomenon occurs largely because of the body's return to homeostasis (a state of equilibrium in the body) which gives the runner a sense of euphoria where they sometimes describe the feeling is that they could go on forever. This is in stark contrast to the first few minutes of exercise where the runner feels as if they will collapse if they continue. The fact is that absent this complex and miraculous process, extended rigorous exercise would cause us to collapse. The process described above is an essential part of healthy vascular function.

In response to pathogens which damage this organ (the endothelium), and in response to our failure to properly utilize this system via regular exercise, the endothelium begins to be compromised. This compromise is reflected and can often be measured and monitored via vascular function testing.

Most of us know and understand this intuitively and intrinsically if we have ever gone for an extended period without rigorous exercise followed by an attempt to restart a program of rigorous exercise. In addition to the inevitable muscular atrophy we can expect to feel in every muscle of our body, we also lose vascular function both from failure to use, but also from the abuse an unhealthy lifestyle imposes on this critical organ. We feel this in the muscles of our body, we feel it in our inability to 'catch our breath', and we feel it in the muscle myalgia (achiness) we experience immediately following our initial efforts to restart our exercise program. An important piece of our ability to exercise effectively is this often misunderstood but crucial vascular function.

Rather than address each of the functional tests below (which would probably result in another book) we will talk about a couple of the more popular tests – and then contrast them briefly to a few of the other vascular function tests we have already discussed.

As mentioned earlier, high blood sugar, high insulin, cigarette smoke, and other sources of inflammation damage the intima. The goal of most vascular function testing is to measure damage to the intima which includes the endothelium – a key component of vascular function with an eye towards making changes necessary to effect improvement. Ongoing vascular function testing provides us the evidence that our intervention has been effective.

ABI (ANKLE BRACHIAL INDEX) –
A VASCULAR FUNCTION TEST

DEFINITION

The Ankle-Brachial pressure Index (ABI or ABPI) is the ratio of the highest blood pressure in either the right or left ankles divided by the highest blood pressure of the corresponding arm (brachial). Lower ankle pressures (<.9) suggests that there is lower vascular function which could be due to plaque blocking the arteries to the legs, but also could be due to other conditions common in diabetics and other patients with other means of vascular compromise.

The concept appears simple, but ABI requires good quality systems. The test is simple, inexpensive, and can be completed in just a few minutes. The test is similar to a blood pressure test, but more involved.

Blood pressure cuffs are placed on each arm (both left and right) where the highest systolic blood pressures are then measured using plethsymography. Following the measurement of the brachial (arm) blood pressures, cuffs are placed on each leg (ankle) and once again the highest systolic blood pressures for each ankle are measured. In a clinical environment, ultrasound is often used to get a more accurate read of the systolic and diastolic start and ending points. Waveform ultrasound images are also taken and analyzed.

A calculation is then made to compare and calculate the difference between the highest pressure seen on either ankle divided by those found on the corresponding arms (the brachial). The ratio determines the patient's ankle-brachial indexes and the lowest of the two indexes correlates to each patient's relative risk for CV disease, heart attack and/or stroke.

The ABI test is not specific (a term which refers to the number of people without disease who test negative – the higher the specificity, the more accurate and useful the test), but it's worthwhile because it assesses a separate vascular bed from the coronary and carotid arteries. It is also unique in that it provides some assessment as to the elasticity and function of the arteries. In a clinical setting, the technician or physician administering the test may have the patient perform some modest exercise such as toe lifts prior to taking these measurements. This provides additional complexity and specificity to the test results which can enhance the usefulness or predictive value of the test.

BACKGROUND

Scientific evidence indicates that ABI is a valid and worthwhile measurement. Although you could do it at home, we do not recommend relying on the results of a home reading. The provider must focus on technique, reproducibility, and clinical relevance. Because of these concerns, we recommend that all but the largest clinics consider outsourcing ABI, CIMT, and functional vascular testing to a provider with robust quality structures, systems, and processes for these tests. With the ABI, for example, this includes using ultrasound and pressure waveform analysis to further refine the measurements. These are not available at most homes or small clinics.

ABI WORKSHEET

Ankle-Brachial Index Interpretation
Above 0.90: Normal
0.71 - 0.90: Mild Obstruction
0.41 - 0.70: Moderate Obstruction
0.00 - 0.40: Severe Obstruction

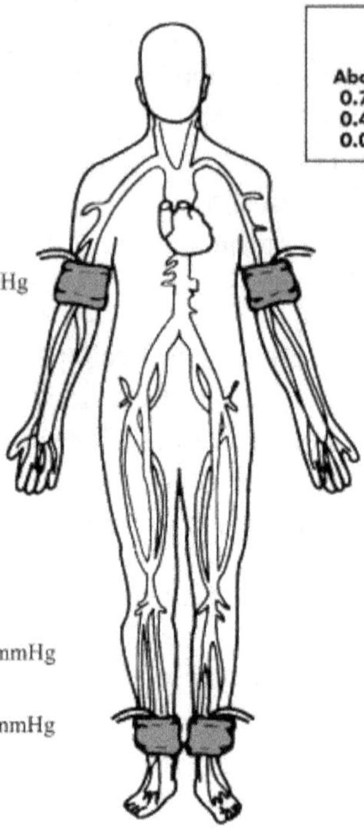

Right Arm:
Systolic Pressure [| |] mmHg

Left Arm:
Systolic Pressure [| |] mmHg

Right Ankle:
Systolic Pressure
Posterior Tibial (PT) [| |] mmHg
Dorsalis Pedis (DP) [| |] mmHg

Left Ankle:
Systolic Pressure
Posterior Tibial (PT) [| |] mmHg
Dorsalis Pedis (DP) [| |] mmHg

Right ABI equals Ratio of:
Higher of the Right Ankle Pressures (PT or DP) [| |] mmHg
Higher Arm Pressure (right or left arm) [| |] mmHg
= [ ].[|] *

Left ABI equals Ratio of:
Higher of the Left Ankle Pressures (PT or DP) [| |] mmHg
Higher Arm Pressure (right or left arm) [| |] mmHg
= [ ].[|] *

* The lower of these numbers is the patient's overall ABI.
Overall ABI (lower ABI) = ____________

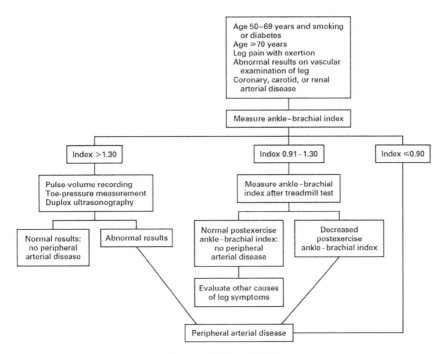

Source: (Hiatt, 2001)

An ABI result of ≤ 0.90 increases the lifetime odds of having a heart attack and stroke by as much as 400% (Khan, 2008), (Diehm, 2004). The sensitivity (the test's ability to correctly detect patients with disease or with a particular condition) of this test is >95%, and the specificity (the test's ability to accurately identify those patients without the disease) is also >95% (Khan, 2008). This sensitivity and specificity, however, assume technical proficiency when administering and interpreting the results. A great deal of variability is shown in other studies where the technicians performing the exam were not trained to administer the test correctly. (Feigelson HS, 1994). When performed by an untrained person, the sensitivity and specificity can drop below 40%. That is a significant difference, which explains why many healthcare providers may be reluctant to use it in their practices. They may have even had an experience where the test contradicted their other testing measures. We recommend leaving ABI to the experts.

Peripheral Arterial Disease (PAD)

PAD is a general term meaning significant blockage of arteries outside the chest and brain. It can result in pain, loss of function of the limb, or even amputation. At least 8 million Americans have it. The presence of PAD is a significant risk factor for coronary artery disease, and significantly increases the future risk of heart attack or stroke. (Murabito, 2003), (Zheng, 1997) For example, Medicare Advantage has an HCC (Hierachical Condition Category) adjustment factor of 0.299 for PAD. That means that Medicare expects to spend about a third more on medical care for people with documented vascular disease.

As mentioned before, plaque reflects a systemic disease process and not a local condition. This means if some arteries have plaque, it is most likely that all or most of the arterial beds do. Plaque is not just found in a single location. If plaque is found in one arterial bed, it will most likely be found in all of them. Similar to the plaque on your teeth, if your dentist only cleaned the plaque or tarter on a single tooth, you would probably look for another dentist. Dental plaque is systemic to the entire mouth. Dental plaque found on the front of the incisors means it will most likely also be found behind the molars.

The same is true for our circulatory system. The conditions that exist in the 3 inches or so of a vessel wall measured in an average IMT exam, also exist in nearly all the nearly 100,000 miles of vessels in the average adult.

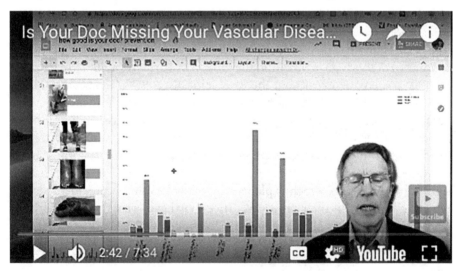

Source: Ford Brewer's YouTube Channel

Arterial plaque is known to indicate an increased risk of heart attack and stroke. Functional testing provides additional insight to what is going on in these vessels.

Why is it that providers do not use the ABI and other functional tests more often? We provided an explanation. We have also provided the science supporting its use as a screening tool. For many clinics, functional testing can be a great addition to biomarkers and structural testing like the ones described in this book.

JACK'S STORY

Jack was a 46-year-old professor at a major university when we first met. His day consisted of a lecture or two, and many more hours sitting in his office speaking to students or other faculty members and reading periodicals. He also spent a fair amount of time watching educational videos. Jack's exercise consisted almost entirely of occasional walks across the university campus to conduct business or to speak with other faculty or administrative members. These were occurring with less and less frequency.

Both of Jack's parents died prematurely (before the age of 70) from heart disease so he had a fair amount of concern about having a heart attack and stroke and not living long enough to see his 3 children's children. Jack stood at 5'8' and he weighed 210lbs when he first came to us. This suggested he was obese and very nearly morbidly obese. He was 'stout' and his belly measured 43', which strongly suggested he was insulin resistant and prediabetic.

Jack had heard about CardioRisk from a friend who recommended he get a few tests to assuage his concerns about heart disease. We administered a CIMT and an ABI on Jack on his first visit. Jack's CIMT exam revealed a small plaque measuring 1.4mm in his right carotid artery and he had enough inflammation in his artery to make him equivalent to someone who was > 80 years of age. Jack's ABI measured 0.9 which is right on the boarder for abnormal. Given the plaque in his artery, we suggested he probably also should tell his physician to look for pre-diabetes, which often results in peripheral artery disease. Jack was heading very quickly towards a heart attack or stroke.

The visual evidence of plaque in his artery, combined with the functional measurement showing vascular disease in his extremities provided Jack the motivation he needed to get on a program. Jack showed his results to his primary care physician who was unfamiliar with these technologies but took the time to call us to review the science.

The evidence of disease provided Jack's physician with enough evidence to start Jack on a statin, and on pre-diabetes medication, along with an aggressive lifestyle intervention. Jack was disciplined about his carbohydrate intake and used intermittent fasting to help reset his metabolism. He was religious about taking his medications.

Jack showed up the following year to be tested again. We were delighted to find a significant reduction in the amount of inflammation in his arteries. In just one year, Jack's arteries had improved to where they were now equivalent to someone who was 65 years of age. Although he needed to continue to work, this was so exciting for him because it provided him evidence that his intervention was working.

Jack's plaque had gone from soft to heterogenous. This meant that it was stabilizing and posed a much lower risk of rupturing and causing a future event. Finally, Jack's ABI also showed improvement to an index of 1.1. The empirical evidence provided by the CIMT and ABI exam gave Jack motivation, not just to attack it for a week – but he remains active and focused on his heart health.

We have now watched Jack for over 5 years. We have seen his weight decrease by more than 40 lbs. Jack's belly circumference is now 36 . . . a 7 inch change from where he started. Jack's plaque is now completely echogenic or hardened so there is very little chance it will ever rupture or erode. Jack's arterial age has decreased to 60 years of age, which is now much closer to his chronological age and demonstrative of a nearly complete arrest of the inflammation previously in his arteries. Jack's ABI continues to demonstrate a normal index.

Perhaps most important is that Jack feels so much better. He feels good enough to maintain a rigorous daily exercise routine. Jack reports that maintaining a healthy diet 'just feels better' and that his joints no longer ache. Jack reported that he is more sexually active and that he feels better about his own body image. He feels he delivers his lectures with more energy and enthusiasm and this has resulted in much more positive reviews by the administration and his students. These are the kinds of changes which often occur when patients can visually see their disease and monitor their progress year over year with reliable data.

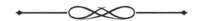

PROBLEMS WITH TESTS

RADIATION: NUCLEAR STRESS TESTS FOLLOWED BY CORONARY ANGIOGRAM FOLLOWED BY STENTS RESULTS IN EXCESS.

Let us review the basics:

- A Sievert is the equivalent dose of radiation exposure multiplied by the absorbed energy, averaged by mass over an organ or tissue of interest by a radiation weighting factor appropriate to the type and energy of the radiation. Sieverts and their micro measurements (e.g. Millisieverts (mSv), and Microsieverts (uSv)) essentially measure the health effect of the ionizing radiation over time.

- There is radiation exposure with Coronary Calcium Scores, CT angiograms, Nuclear Stress Tests, and Coronary Angiogram, as well as with Stents.

- The Sievert expression of the radiation doses are highest in Nuclear Stress Tests (2-12 mSv), invasive Angiograms (8 mSv), and with Stents (15-20 mSv).

- The CT Angiogram emits a radiation dose that is very much a moving target. The dose delivered is reported to have dropped 80% over the past decade (from 12.7 mSv to 2.7 mSv) with new equipment & techniques (McKeown 2018). However, as of 2017, the median dose was still 9.6 mSv (Carpeggiani, 2017).

- The Coronary Calcium Score delivers less than 1 mSv, so it is less of a practical concern for the typical 60-year-old looking for clarity about heart attack risk.

- There is no radiation with CIMT, ABI, or two types of stress tests: exercise EKG and Stress Echo.

- 1 Sievert = 1000 mSv (Millisieverts)

- 1 Millisievert = 1000 uSv (Microsieverts)

- Increased cancer risk from radiation occurs at 100 mSv of **lifetime**, cumulative radiation exposure. (Gilbert, 2010).

- Radiation exposure occurs in nature (sun), from cell phones, from travel in an airplane, from medical testing, and MANY other sources. The cumulative effect of this exposure is what increases a human's lifetime risk of cancer from radiation. See Images on page 132 & 133.

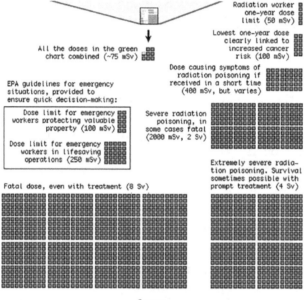

Source:
http://www.nrc.gov/reading-rm/doc-collections/cfr/part020/
http://www.nrc.gov/reading-rm/doc-collections/fact-sheets/tritium-radiation-fs.html
http://www.nema.ne.gov/technological/dose-limits.html
http://www.deq.idaho.gov/inl_oversight/radiation/dose_calculator.cfm
http://www.deq.idaho.gov/inl_oversight/radiation/radiation_guide.cfm
http://mitnse.com/
http://www.mext.go.jp/component/a_menu/other/detail/__icsFiles/afieldfile/2011/03/18/1303727_1716.pdf
http://blog.vornaskotti.com/2010/07/15/into-the-zone-chernobyl-pripyat/
http://dels-old.nas.edu/dels/rpt_briefs/rerf_final.pdf
http://en.wikipedia.org/wiki/Sievert
http://radiology.rsna.org/content/248/1/254
http://webcache.googleusercontent.com/search?q=cache:BK-ukkJ_Fh0J:www.mext.go.jp/english/
radioactivity_level/detail/1304853.htm+http://www.mext.go.jp/english/radioactivity_level/detail/1304853.
htm&cd=1&hl=en&ct=clnk&gl=us&source=www.google.com
http://chottomatte.net/2011/03/16/tokyo-radiation-levels-daily-updates/

Effective Doses for Adults from Various Nuclear Medicine Examinations

Examination*	Effective Dose (mSv)	Administered Activity (MBq)[†]	Effective Dose (mSv/MBq)[‡]
Brain (^{99m}Tc-HMPAO–exametazime)	6.9	740	0.0093
Brain (^{99m}Tc-ECD–Neurolite)	5.7	740	0.0077
Brain (^{18}F-FDG)	14.1	740	0.019
Thyroid scan (sodium iodine 123)	1.9	25	0.075 (15% uptake)
Thyroid scan (^{99m}Tc-pertechnetate)	4.8	370	0.013
Parathyroid scan (^{99m}Tc-sestamibi)	6.7	740	0.009
Cardiac stress-rest test (thallium 201 chloride)	40.7	185	0.22
Cardiac rest-stress test (^{99m}Tc-sestamibi 1-day protocol)	9.4	1100	0.0085 (0.0079 stress, 0.0090 rest)
Cardiac rest-stress test (^{99m}Tc-sestamibi 2-day protocol)	12.8	1500	0.0085 (0.0079 stress, 0.0090 rest)
Cardiac rest-stress test (Tc-tetrofosmin)	11.4	1500	0.0076
Cardiac ventriculography (^{99m}Tc-labeled red blood cells)	7.8	1110	0.007
Cardiac (^{18}F-FDG)	14.1	740	0.019
Lung perfusion (^{99m}Tc-MAA)	2.0	185	0.011
Lung ventilation (xenon 133)	0.5	740	0.00074
Lung ventilation (^{99m}Tc-DTPA)	0.2	1300 (40 actually inhaled)	0.0049
Liver-spleen (^{99m}Tc-sulfur colloid)	2.1	222	0.0094
Biliary tract (^{99m}Tc-disofenin)	3.1	185	0.017
Gastrointestinal bleeding (^{99m}Tc-labeled red blood cells)	7.8	1110	0.007
Gastrointestinal emptying (^{99m}Tc-labeled solids)	0.4	14.8	0.024
Renal (^{99m}Tc-DTPA)	1.8	370	0.0049
Renal (^{99m}Tc-MAG3)	2.6	370	0.007
Renal (^{99m}Tc-DMSA)	3.3	370	0.0088
Renal (^{99m}Tc-glucoheptonate)	2.0	370	0.0054
Bone (^{99m}Tc-MDP)	6.3	1110	0.0057
Gallium 67 citrate	15	150	0.100
Pentreotide (^{111}In)	12	222	0.054
White blood cells (^{99m}Tc)	8.1	740	0.011
White blood cells (^{111}In)	6.7	18.5	0.360
Tumor (^{18}F-FDG)	14.1	740	0.019

* DMSA = dimercaptosuccinic acid, DTPA = diethylenetriaminepentaacetic acid, ECD = ethyl cysteinate dimer, ^{18}F = fluorine 18, FDG = fluorodeoxyglucose, HMPAO = hexamethylpropyleneamine oxime, ^{111}In = indium 111, MAA = macroaggregated albumin, MAG3 = mercaptoacetyltriglycine, MDP = methylene diphosphonate, ^{99m}Tc = technetium 99m.

[†] Recommended ranges vary, although most laboratories tend to use the upper end of suggested ranges.

[‡] From reference 74.

(Mettler, 2008)

BACKGROUND

Nuclear stress tests account for 10% of the ionizing radiation exposure of the population in the US. (National Council on Radiation Protection and Measurements 2006) Nuclear stress tests involve radiation equivalent to approximately 400 chest X-rays.

The risk of death and disability from a heart attack is significantly greater than the risk of death from radiation exposure for patients with significant risk. Not all patients have that much CV risk. That is why you do not see nuclear stress tests routinely performed on teenagers. You also do not see studies where Coronary Calcium Scores are done on populations of healthy youth or children. Caution should be used before deciding to have any procedure which exposes a patient to unnecessary radiation. This should include considering the age of the patient as well as their relative risk of heart attack or stroke compared to the increased risk of cancer from radiation exposure.

RADIOACTIVE COMBINATION: NUCLEAR STRESS TEST FOLLOWED BY ANGIOGRAPHY AND STENTS

Catheter coronary angiograms still represent one of the highest X-ray and radiation exposures of all medical examinations (surpassed only by stent placements in the CV space). Radiation doses for coronary angiograms have not changed significantly over the years. It is important to recognize that newer equipment generally emits smaller doses of radiation. Older equipment may still emit unacceptable levels of radiation, especially when performed in sequence with other radiological exams. A great deal of variation, in terms of radiological exposure, occurs between the equipment and protocol used by the facility performing the exam.

The biggest concern over radiation exposure occurs when a combination of nuclear stress tests are followed by angiograms, which are then followed by one or more stents. In PCI procedures (percutaneous intervention), multiple radiological procedures are commonly performed in succession. When this combination is repeated multiple times, the radiation risk becomes significant. This happens more than you might think. The problem is confounded by the fact that routine radiation safety procedures are often ignored, especially in the US, as we will see in the next section.

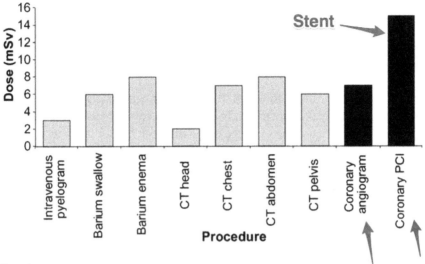

Figure 1

Relative patient effective dose for medical imaging procedures. Typical doses for medical imaging procedures. Adapted from data from Mettler et al.7 mSv, millisievert; CT, computed tomography; PCI, percutaneous coronary intervention.

(Mettler, 2008)

IGNORING ROUTINE RADIATION SAFETY GUIDELINES

As mentioned elsewhere, most medical standards committees warn against the current practice of overutilization of stress tests, angiogram, and stents. Even when the imaging is done according to standards, it is not done with a focus on minimizing radiation. A study of practice conducted by the International Atomic Energy Agency (IAEA) demonstrated significant variations in radiation doses and in the use of best practices that can help to reduce dose, among laboratories worldwide. (Einstein, 2015). Two studies published in JAMA Internal Medicine demonstrated unnecessary radiation exposure from cardiac imaging. (Mercuri, 2016) (Mercuri M. P., 2016)

What we learned from these studies is that even in instances when nuclear stress tests seem indicated, patients are likely to get too much radiation. In a study of 308 nuclear cardiology laboratories in 65 countries, the authors compared radiation exposure among U.S. patients with their peers in other countries. The investigators found that U.S. patients receive a surprising 20% more radiation than their peers abroad. The difference was, in part, explained by the lack of necessary radiation safety procedures (weight-based dosing and judicious use of technetium Tc99m).

Another factor is the order in which the cardiac imaging is performed. When a stress imaging study is abnormal, it is essential to compare it to a resting study to rule out alternative causes for the abnormal test results (such as scars and artifact). But if the stress imaging is normal, the resting image (which requires additional radiation) is unnecessary -- and it is a source of unneeded radiation. Stress imaging, therefore, should generally be performed first, and a resting study obtained only if the stress imaging test is abnormal. (Mercuri 2016)

Remarkably, this is just the opposite of what usually happens in the U.S. According to a second study, rest imaging is performed first more than 90% of the time; in Europe, rest imaging is ordered first 16% of the time. It probably won't come as a surprise to learn that financial incentives make it more profitable to perform both resting and stress imaging rather than a stress imaging test alone.

RADIATION AND THE CORONARY CALCIUM SCORE

Let us begin by putting the radiation from Coronary Calcium Scores in perspective. The radiation dose from each of those 8 million nuclear stress tests done annually is over 10 times the radiation dose from a single Coronary Calcium Score.

The Coronary Calcium Score uses C.T. technology. That means there is radiation. Newer X-ray imaging equipment continues to decrease the amount of radiation exposure, but it is still there. Radiation risk is the reason that average Coronary Calcium Score tables do not exist for young, healthy populations. Review committees for studies involving Human subjects (research ethics) would never agree to radiate healthy people just to document their Coronary Calcium Scores. With CIMT, on the other hand, the research has been completed, which provides epidemiological average measurements for healthy subjects of all ages. CIMT uses ultrasound, so there is no ionizing radiation risk involved.

The risk of cancer from radiation exposure is minimal for Coronary Calcium Score technology compared to the alternatives and in the context of middle-aged adults. The lifetime radiation cancer risk from a Coronary Calcium Score is about 1% (due to a dose of about one mJ millijoule). But this is in a newborn, not in a 50 or 60-year-old. People getting a Coronary Calcium Score usually need to know if their risk of a heart attack or stroke over the next ten years is closer to 5% or 25%. Most agree that the CAC radiation risk is worth that critical information.

There has been some debate regarding how much radiation is routinely involved. It is improving each year. Initially the exposure was between 2 and 10 mSv (millisievert, the amount of radiation absorbed by the body). A recent study of this radiation exposure was nested within the well-known MESA study. It was found on a practical basis to be closer to 1 mSv (millisievert). (Messenger, 2016).

Even the earlier, higher radiation risk estimates are not that high compared to the risk of heart attack demonstrated by the study. The lifetime risk of cancer in the previous groups (2 to 10 mJ exposure) was estimated to be 1-in-1,000 lifetime risk. (Lifetime refers to an infant's lifetime. That same dose has far less chance to result in cancer death in a 60-year-old with CV risk). Since the risk of heart attack and stroke with untreated plaque is 40%-81% in just ten years (Belcaro, 2001), the addition of .1% risk of cancer from radiation is acceptable for most.

Overutilization: did we mention stress tests and cardiac catheter angiograms are overutilized?

RUNAWAY HEALTHCARE INFLATION: THE HUMAN ATM

The US fails to control surgical and medical procedure utilization. You do not have to be a doctor or a medical economist to know that. Atul Gawande, MD, moved this discussion to center stage 10 years ago, starting with his article "The Cost Conundrum" (Gawande, 2009). He did not say that all doctors practice medicine for financial gain; just a lot of them. That is enough to drive runaway healthcare costs. In the 10 years since Gawande's article in The New Yorker, this situation has become much worse. Neither insurance nor government control of healthcare has been popular or effective at controlling the cost or quality of these procedures.

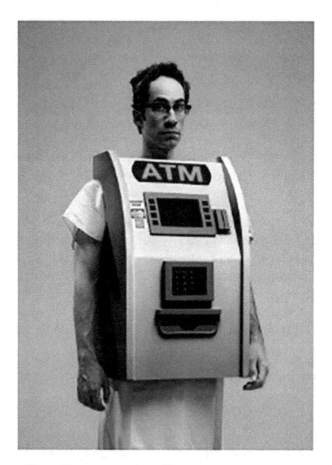

Costlier care is often worse care.

Photograph by Phillip Toledano

(From Gawande 2009)

Even a decade ago, almost half (43%) of primary care physicians believed that much of the provided healthcare is unnecessary, according to a study in the Archives of Internal Medicine. The physicians point to other physicians (and themselves to a much lesser extent) as the ones responsible for unnecessary care. Only 28% said that they personally were testing and referring more than the ideal. 76% blamed the practice on malpractice concerns. 83% thought they could be sued for not ordering a test, but only 21% thought they could be sued for ordering an unnecessary test. Over half (52%) said they were ordering tests due to performance measures in their contracts. 40% said it was due to a lack of time. Over one third (39%) believed other primary care physicians would order fewer diagnostic tests if those tests did not generate extra income. Almost two thirds (62%) said specialists were ordering tests due to financial incentives. These physicians said 10% of the patients they see each day do not need it. 95% said that doctors vary in the testing and treatment choices for similar patients (Sirovich, 2011).

Physicians as a group are not alone in stating there is much waste in medical care. The NAM (National Academy of Medicine - formerly the IOM, or Institute of Medicine) said in 2010 that if prices had grown as quickly as healthcare, a gallon of milk would cost $48 (Yong, 2010).

OVERUSE OF STRESS TESTS

2014 and 2015 were big years for waking up to the fact that we do too many stress tests. The New York Times published an article by pediatrician Nikolas Bakalar titled 'Too Much Cardiac Testing'.

"There is no evidence that stress tests, electrocardiograms or myocardial perfusion imaging (the so-called nuclear stress test that involves exposure to radiation) have any advantages over routine risk assessment in asymptomatic people. All the tests commonly produce false positives that lead to further unnecessary testing, and all involve extra expense." Bakalar was quoting a new guideline from the American College of Physicians. Bakalar further quoted the author of the guidelines article (Chou) as saying, "doing a stress test doesn't give you extra information that is helpful" in an asymptomatic person (Bakalar, March 16, 2015) (Chou, 2015). Chou chose strong words. Yet he did it as a spokesman for America's internists.

A 2014 study in the Annals of Internal Medicine stated that over one third (at least 34.6%) of nuclear stress tests are inappropriate. That same study linked a price tag of over half a billion dollars ($501million) to the unnecessary tests. Simple estimates (2.7 million nuclear stress test times $630/test) indicate it may be at least three times that amount (Ladapo, 2014). Medical boards, professional associations, and foundations have developed their own efforts to help. For example, the ABIM (American Board of Internal Medicine) joined forces with Consumer Reports to inform the American public about the dangers and costs of physician-driven over-testing. They cite the Consumer Reports study indicating that 44% of asymptomatic adults age 40 to 60 had unnecessary stress tests.

More recently, in 2019, the problem continued with no end in sight (Gluckman, 2019).

ARE NUCLEAR STRESS TESTS REALLY USED FOR MORE COMPLICATED TESTS?

The plethora of stress tests performed annually shows that many patients and their doctors assume they will get more value than cost out of the study. Let us give stress tests their due; there is some predictive value, especially for patients that reach a very high level of exercise intensity. Given the fact that the average cost range for a stress EKG is $200 to 300 and for a Nuclear Stress Tests the average is 3 to 4 times that, you might expect to see many more Stress EKGs. The higher cost of Nuclear Stress Tests suggests they would be indicated for far more complicated cases.

However, on average, simple Stress EKG's account for only around 10% of the total number of Stress Tests. The vast majority of Stress Tests completed in the US are variations of Nuclear Stress Tests (Stress using MRI, or Stress SPECT imaging). Despite being the least expensive, Stress EKG is just not very popular anymore. The reasons should be obvious. It is clear that a stress EKG doesn't accomplish much in terms of ensuring future health, as we saw in cases like Tim Russert's. The perception is that Nuclear Stress Tests are much better. They are not!

Dr. Marty Makary of Johns Hopkins studied this concept in 2016. He found that roughly one-quarter of physicians ordered Nuclear Stress Tests less than

25% of the time. About 40% of physicians ordered Nuclear Stress Tests over half the time. 10% of physicians ordered Nuclear Stress Tests over 75% of the time. Yes, and some docs ordered Nuclear Stress Tests 100% of the time (Gluckman, 2019).

COST OF STRESS TESTS

Doctors usually think of stress tests as inexpensive. For the purposes of this chapter, we will refer to a few websites. Here is what they report:

- Choosingwisely.org: $175 or more. (Referring to stress ekg)

- Mdsave.com: The national average is $891.

- Healthcarebluebook.com: $160 to $606 for fair price estimates.

- Abcnews.go.com: $200 for a basic Stress Test, with an average of $630 for Nuclear Stress Tests.

- Health.costhelper.com: Patients with medical insurance covering a portion of the cost of the Stress Test procedure can expect to pay $200-$400 total out of their pockets, depending on the patients' copay responsibility.

- Harvard Pilgrim Health Care (Harvardpilgrim.org): Members are charged $270-$379 for the test itself and an additional $24- $39 for an interpretation of the test. Uninsured patients will likely pay $1,000-$5,000 for a Stress Test and the required analysis.

SPECT AND PET MACHINE & PROGRAM COSTS

According to multiple studies, SPECT and PET scan Stress Tests have the highest sensitivity and specificity and they are the most expensive. That is because the technology is expensive. New machines can cost in excess of $ 2M. Refurbished systems can cost around $350k. Upkeep and maintenance can be as much as $100k /year. The radiologic tracer can cost around $40k /month. These numbers do not include compliance or staffing. These costs make is cost prohibitive to nearly everyone, unless there is scale (e.g. there are many people getting these tests). It is important to remember that even these higher technology tests still perform at low sensitivity and specificity.

WHAT ABOUT OVERUSE OF STENTS?

The COURAGE trial of 2007 and ORBITA trial of 2018 are just two of the multiple studies that demonstrate stents do not prevent heart attacks. AE Carroll, a pediatrician, and reporter for the New York Times, covered these studies and more. He blamed the continued popularity of stents on the placebo effect (Carroll A. , 2018).

MEDICAL BOARDS, RESEARCHERS, AND THE PRESS AGREE – STENTS OVERUSED.

The ACC (American College of Cardiology) teamed with Choosing Wisely®, an affiliate of the ABIM (American Board of Internal Medicine) Foundation. One of their goals is to discourage the practice of unnecessary Stent placement.

CHOOSING WISELY

Choosing Wisely "is an organization whose stated mission is to promote conversations between clinicians and patients by helping patients choose care that is:

- Supported by the evidence
- Not duplicative of other tests or procedures already received
- Free from harm
- Truly necessary

In 2012, national organizations representing medical specialists started asking their members to identify tests or procedures commonly used in their field, whose necessity should be questioned and discussed. This call to action has resulted in specialty-specific "Lists of Things Providers and Patients Should Question." (Choosing Wisely®, Our Mission, https://www.choosingwisely.org/our-mission)

The ACC/Choosing Wisely Top 5 in Cardiology

Here are the top 5 situations in which the ACC has discouraged current overuse:

Avoid performing stress cardiac imaging or advanced non-invasive imaging in the initial evaluation of patients without cardiac symptoms unless high-risk markers are present.

Asymptomatic, low-risk patients account for up to 45 percent of unnecessary "screening." Testing should be performed only when the following findings are present: diabetes in patients older than 40-years-old; peripheral arterial disease; or greater than 2 percent yearly risk for coronary heart disease events.

 Avoid performing annual stress cardiac imaging or advanced non-invasive imaging as part of routine follow-up in asymptomatic patients.

Performing stress cardiac imaging or advanced non-invasive imaging in patients without symptoms on a serial or scheduled pattern (e.g., every one to two years or at a heart procedure anniversary) rarely results in any meaningful change in patient management. This practice may, in fact, lead to unnecessary invasive procedures and excess radiation exposure without any proven impact on patients' outcomes. Exceptions to this rule include patients more than five years after a bypass operation, more than 2 years after a stenting procedure, or after having a stent placed in the left main coronary artery.

 Avoid performing stress cardiac imaging or advanced non-invasive imaging as a pre-operative assessment in patients scheduled to undergo low-risk non-cardiac surgery.

Non-invasive testing is not useful for patients undergoing low-risk non-cardiac surgery (that is, with a <1% combined clinical/surgical perioperative risk of myocardial infarction or death, e.g., cataract removal, endoscopy). These types of tests do not change the patient's clinical management or outcomes and could result in increased costs and unnecessary downstream procedures.

Avoid performing echocardiography as routine follow-up for mild, asymptomatic native valve disease in adult patients with no change in signs or symptoms.

Patients with native valve disease usually have years without symptoms before the onset of deterioration. An echocardiogram is not recommended yearly unless there is a change in clinical status.

 Avoid performing routine electrocardiography (ECG) screening as part of pre-operative or pre-procedural evaluations for asymptomatic patients undergoing low-risk surgical procedures.

Despite potential value in having a pre-operative ECG to identify unsuspected cardiac abnormalities or as a comparison after a perioperative event, the likelihood of benefit for patients at low (<1%) risk of major cardiovascular events (death or myocardial infarction) is very small. Unnecessary ECGs can lead to needless consults, delays and changes to operative plans, which may counterbalance any potential benefit for the patient. In the absence of scientific studies establishing the value of a pre-operative ECG in a low cardiovascular risk population, the routine ordering of pre-operative ECGs prior to low-risk procedures should be discouraged.

Source: https://www.choosingwisely.org/societies/american-college-of-cardiology/

DILEMMAS: LOGICAL, THERAPEUTIC, FINANCIAL, AND ETHICAL

If you are a physician, what are you supposed to say to those patients coming through your door? They are sitting in your waiting room. They are waiting to tell you that their uncle just had a fatal heart attack, and they want you to make sure they do not have a similar problem. They have worried about it . . . a lot. If they can pass a Stress Test, isn't that the best assurance they do not have a CV risk problem? They do not know what we have just covered in this book. Unfortunately, too many doctors are unfamiliar with this information as well.

Patients have expectations, and doctors attempt to meet those expectations. For many physicians, it is not just the financial concern of losing patients. Doctors went into medicine with a desire to help people. These physicians want to make their patients healthy and happy. If they cannot do both, they will often take one or the other.

Since there is also a major lack of appreciation or knowledge among physicians and patients about other screening tools (CIMT, Coronary Calcium Score, and CT angiograms), the result is a gross overuse of the more obvious or common tests - the Stress Tests. This problem of potential serious illness and the supposed lack of solutions leads to additional financial and ethical dilemmas. It is a trap for medical overuse. That is why this one condition (heart disease) is estimated to cost the American public $1.2 Trillion annually by the year 2030. That is a BIG number. Most of us do not deal with numbers with that many zeros in it but let us try to put those costs into perspective.

At the time of this book's publishing, there were approximately 500,000 homeless people in the US. Also, there are approximately 20,000,000 adults currently registered for college. $1.2Trillion dollars could buy EVERY homeless person in America a home valued at $2.4 Million and that is just with the FIRST year's savings. Each year (assuming we could implement the savings from heart disease each year) we could write a check to EVERY person registered for college in the amount of $60,000 for their tuition and annual expenses.

We want to put these dollars into a perspective we can all understand. They are BIG numbers. It is easy to lose sight of them when someone rattles off a large deficit, governmental spending-sized number like a Trillion dollars . . . but these number are REAL!

TEST CHARACTERISTICS: FALSE POSITIVE AND FALSE NEGATIVE TEST RESULTS

We think of lab and imaging tests as objective, correct, and reliable. This is an overestimate of the facts.

IS THE TEST DESIGNED FOR ITS CURRENT USE?

Before discussing the confusing world of test sensitivity, specificity, and predictive value statistics, it is probably important to examine a more critical issue. This issue is so obvious that it usually passes without notice. The issue is this: Does the intended use of a test match the design of the test? The stress test is a good test to measure cardiac conditioning. The design of this test does not really match its intended purpose when attempting to use it to identify a person's risk of future heart attack and/or stroke. It does not work for the actual mechanism of a heart attack. That is because it does not measure the risk of a soft plaque bursting and forming a clot. It just measures blood flow. When used for the wrong purpose, a test's formal sensitivity and specificity statistics do not matter.

Let us consider an application to everyday realities. One must consider the intended purpose of any test before deciding to use it. For instance, if the intended use of Russert's Stress Test were to predict a future heart attack, it was used incorrectly, and it yielded an incorrect result (a false negative). It also failed to predict sudden death related to a heart attack. If the purpose of Russert's test were to detect plaque, it also failed. Russert already knew he had plaque pursuant to his positive Coronary Calcium Score. If the goal were to measure conditioning, Russert's test was right. His exercise tolerance was good - until it was not . . . and he died.

SENSITIVITY AND SPECIFICITY

There are technical terms for medical tests describing how often the results are right - or wrong. The sensitivity of a test is the percentage of times it would correctly identify a person with disease in a population made up entirely of people with the disease (true positive rate).

Specificity is the percentage of times a test would identify those without the disease (the true negative rate) in a population of people without the disease.

Sensitivity and specificity are not the same, by the way, and these concepts can get confusing.

Sensitivity and specificity are technical terms which also help to describe the relative value of screening tests. Although these can get statistically complicated, this is a book for the public, not medical testing epidemiologists. We will only discuss what is necessary to understand in order to make the best choice of tests for your own situation.

These testing characteristics lead to the problems we have repeated throughout this book. A false negative stress test incorrectly gave Tim Russert (and his provider/physician) an excuse to delay his weight loss, which was ultimately fatal. It minimized the urgency of the matter. The problem is that there are a lot of false-negative stress tests when using these tests to predict one's risk of impending or future heart attack or stroke. The opposite (false-positives) are also common, and these results lead to an unwelcome and unnecessary trip to the catheter lab.

THE DIFFERENCE BETWEEN HIGH AND LOW-RISK POPULATIONS

Sensitivity and specificity drive another concept: PVP (Predictive Value of a Positive). Here is the simple version of this concept. The same Stress Tests will yield different results and predictive values depending on the risk of the patient (or portion of the population with the disease). For example: if 100 low-risk teenagers and 100 high-risk 65-year-old patients are submitted to Stress Tests, the test results will be significantly different between the two groups.

In this scenario, for example, a positive stress test in the teen group is likely to be a false positive. A positive stress test in the older, higher-risk population is more likely to be a true positive. That difference is driven by the portion of the population with the disease. The probability of a true positive (that a positive test result accurately demonstrates true disease in the patient) actually depends on the percentage of the population with true disease. In the example just stated, the PVP (Predictive Value of a Positive) is higher in the older, sicker population.

After getting past the mental/logical gymnastics of lab test characteristics, the usefulness of a particular test boils down to one practical fact. None of the standards committees recommend stress tests for low-risk individuals of any age. They know that positive tests are much more likely to be false positives and they all agree that too many tests are being performed on populations that will result in more false positive results.

Sensitivity and Specificity of the Different Types of Stress Tests

Let us look at the often-quoted superiority of the Nuclear Stress Test. The sensitivity and specificity of Nuclear and Echo Stress Tests are better than that of the Stress EKG, at least as demonstrated in most peer-reviewed studies. Most doctors can tell you that, even if they cannot define sensitivity and specificity. A meta-analysis (a retrospective review of multiple completed studies on a specific topic) published in the Annals of Internal Medicine suggested the following sensitivity and specificity results (respectively) (Garber 1999):

- Exercise (or stress) EKG: 68% and 77 % in 132 studies of over 24,000 patients.

- Stress echo: 76% and 88% in 6 studies of 510 patients.

- Nuclear stress test: 79% and 73% in 6 studies of 510 patients.

- SPECT MPI: 88% and 77% in 10 studies of 1,174 patients.

- PET scan stress tests: 91% and 82% in 3 studies of 206 patients.

As mentioned previously, formal sensitivity and specificity measurements depend on the targeted populations in the study. The comparison used as the "true north" or "gold standard" for the presence of disease is directly relevant to the stated sensitivity and specificity rates attributed to the particular technology or methodology. A typical comparison used to define the presence of the disease is a plaque on a coronary angiogram. Plaque on a coronary angiogram, however, does not predict heart attacks either. Arbab-Zedah looked at the probability of heart attacks after each type of Stress Test. (Arbab-Zadeh, 2012) see image on page 149.

Table 2

Annualized rates of myocardial infarction and cardiac death at follow up according to stress testing results.

Test	N	Median follow up (months)	MI/Cardiac death with normal test [*]	MI/Cardiac death with abnormal test [°]
Exercise treadmill test	1,647	30	0.80	2.00
Exercise Nuclear MPI	9,930	20	0.65	4.30
Pharmacologic Nuclear MPI	4,988	22	1.78	9.98
Exercise Echocardiography	4,347	36	0.50	2.06
Dobutamine Echocardiography	1,930	32	1.13	4.33

MI, myocardial infarction; MPI, myocardial perfusion imaging.

[*] indicates low risk Duke treadmill score;
[°] indicates high risk Duke treadmill score.

(Arbab-Zadeh, 2012)

If you think that those numbers are not bad, multiply them out to ten-year rates. These are ten-year event rates of 5% to 18% for those with negative Stress Test scores. Those with positive Stress Test scores extrapolate to a 20%-100% ten-year event rate. These numbers demonstrate that Stress Tests indicate a difference in prognosis; but reliance on either a negative or positive Stress Test for the next course of treatment is dangerous.

Also, most heart attack cases did not have a Stress Test just before their heart attack. Because of this fact, they are not included in published sensitivity/specificity statistics. Yet, we know their level of occlusion (2/3 or 68% had less than 50% occlusion just prior to their event) as determined in their autopsy.

DOES NUCLEAR STRESS TESTING RESULT IN A LONGER LIFE?

Does the value of Stress Tests lie in their ability to improve patient survival? Although that seems logical, few studies have used this as an outcome. Garber and Solomon did. They found only seven days of difference between the life expectancy predicted between the various types of Stress Tests. The choice of

Stress Test made virtually no difference in life expectancy. If that is true, what is the real difference - or the value of a Stress EKG vs. a Nuclear Stress Test? The answer . . . none! (Garber 1999)

SURVIVAL AFTER CTA

The SCOT-HEART and PROMISE trials have shown people survive longer after CT Angiograph than after Stress Tests.

So, when your doctor recommends a stress test, stop, and refer to this book.

Test\characteristics	# Completed in the US/year	Cost	Advantages	Disadvantages	Radiation
Stress EKG		$75-$350	Easy access	False +/-	none
Stress Echo		$500-$2500	Easy access	Cost, False +/-	none
Nuclear Stress	8M	$400-$ 850	Easy access	Cost, False +/-	4-10 mSv
Stress SPECT/PET Scan	No record	$4,000 - $15,000	Easy access	Cost, plus false +/--	10-15 mSv
Coronary (cath) Angiogram	1M	$4500-$8000	Good access, definitive anatomy	Radiation & other danger/discomfort, cost	2-12 mSv
ABI Ankle Brachial Index		$50 for BP cuff	DIY, easy	False negative	none
CT Angiogram		$1200 - $2500	Good access, definitive anatomy	Soft plaque often not clear	9.6 mSv (can drop to 2.7 mSv with right equipment
Coronary Calcium Score		$100-$400	Good access, good screen	Shows calcium, not hard or soft plaque, not for follow up	<1 – 5 mSv
CIMT		$95-$400	Shows soft plaque,	Poor access, standardization	none

Source: (Carpeggiani, 2017)

THE MEDICAL STANDARDS DEVELOPMENT PROCESS

CIMT has proven its utility in terms of sensitivity, specificity, reproducibility, and its unique ability to be used to monitor the efficacy of any intervention. The key standards committees have failed to interpret key studies critically, which has led to a failure to recommend CIMT for routine use. The decisions of the medical standards committees have resulted in under-utilization of CIMT and over-reliance on Stress Tests.

ADDING BACK THE "NONTRADITIONAL" RISK FACTORS

Should you or your physician follow the US Preventive Services Guidelines relating to Nontraditional Risk Factors? Alternatively, should you consider adding those nontraditional risk factors to your routine CV risk assessment?

Nontraditional Risk Factor assessment include items like hsCRP, other inflammatory markers, homocysteine, CACS, and CIMT. We recommend adding ALL of these "Nontraditional Risk Factors" to your annual assessments.

Why are we comfortable debating with the standards committees? Dr.s Brewer and Eldredge have BOTH worked with the USPSTF at different times and in different roles.

When Dr Brewer ran the Preventive Medicine Residency program at Hopkins, his residents wrote the science literature reviews for the first set of USPSTF guidelines. Getting close to the medical standards development committees provides an understanding of how they work, and when they do not.

Dr. Eldredge presented the CIMT studies and data discussed below to the USPSTF. The meeting was originally set for 15 minutes. It turned into three hours and ballooned to approximately 27 of their scientists. The result of the meeting was a significant change in the USPSTF position. In practical terms, the CIMT recommendation softened from "don't recommend" to "make your own choice."

Having said that, it is important to understand that standards development is a political process. Like all political processes, it is flawed. People typically defer to a recognized expert on a specific topic. Experts are human; they carry their own biases and often their egos are attached to those bias'.

HISTORICAL EXAMPLES: VITAMIN C AND METFORMIN

The medical standards development is far better than it used to be, at least from a speed to change perspective. Recommendations on the use of vitamin C and Metformin are good examples.

It took nearly 200 years from the time of discovery for Vitamin C to become the standard for scurvy prevention. After that, it was routinely stored in the holds of English military ships. (This led to the frequent use of the name "limeys" for British sailors.)

Metformin took nearly 100 years from its discovery until it became the standard treatment for non-insulin-dependent diabetes mellitus (type II diabetes). Today there is no debate among experts about metformin being the first-line choice of medication for this condition.

While the 100 years it took for Metformin to become the standard of care may seem like a long time . . ., it is only half the time it took for vitamin C to become the standard treatment. Recently, it took slightly over 20 years for antibiotic treatment of ulcer disease to become a standard. Estimates today, in the digital age, demonstrate a profoundly improved timeline from discovery to general use (17 years from discovery to general use). Why 17 years? Again, it is not transmitting the information that takes time, it is changing the minds of the experts.

It makes more sense if you think about the process of standards development. An essential part of the process is getting the consensus of appointed experts. Yet, agreement on anything is sufficiently hard to achieve with any group. In many situations, the thing that needs consensus is a breakthrough treatment or diagnostic tool. Who are the people that usually discover those breakthroughs? Often, the person making a technology breakthrough is not someone who sits on the expert panel for the standards committee.

Experts, therefore, must admit that a breakthrough did occur—a discovery that was not usually made by themselves. Emotions, jealousies, and rivalries make things worse, causing further delay in arriving at a consensus decision. While science usually wins in the end, it is almost always a hard-fought battle.

WHY DON'T THE STANDARDS INCLUDE CIMT?

Well, they did. In the year 2000, the American Heart Association's (AHA) expert panel recommended that CIMT be used routinely in asymptomatic patients because it provided additive value to traditional risk assessment. Perhaps the most compelling case for CIMT can be found in a study completed and published clear back in the year 2000.

In the CAFES-CAVE study, the authors followed 10,000 patients for 10 years. At the onset of this landmark study, they chose a population of low-risk individuals (people who had none of the standard risk factors for heart attacks and strokes). This was important to the study because they had these individuals sign waivers which gave their agreement to NOT be treated during the course of the study (for 10 years). This was appropriate because none of these individuals had risk factors that would have otherwise warranted a medical intervention. The authors planned only to monitor these patients using what was at that time a novel technology - an ultrasound scan (carotid and femoral intima-media thickness or CIMT). (Belcaro, 2001).

The results were astounding and have yet to be improved upon. 21% of these patients went on to have a heart attack and/or stroke during the study period of 10 years. Traditional risk factors would have missed ALL of these patients since they were all asymptomatic and had no traditional risk factors. The ultrasound results (CIMT), by contrast, caught 98.6% of the events.

We have already discussed that a catch rate of 98.6% is better than a home pregnancy test. It is unheard of in medical screening procedures. We are simply not aware of another technology in any genre of medicine that can match it in terms of identifying an asymptomatic patient group before the event occurs.

Notwithstanding this incredible finding demonstrated in a large 100,000 person-year study, many of the experts could not bring themselves to embrace this technology.

Other standards committees have either not recommended, or specifically recommended against the testing based largely on their understanding of two meta-analyses studies.

A meta-analysis is a study that looks at many other studies conducted on a particular subject. Meta-analysis papers (also called literature reviews or lit reviews) are systematic reviews regarding the available or published science in a field of study. It makes sense for the standards committees to use meta-analyses. Demand for meta-analyses of scientific niches has grown dramatically. However, things that make sense sometimes do not work as planned. Sometimes, for example, science itself is not what it appears.

THE NOT-SO-OBVIOUS PROBLEMS WITH SCIENCE: THEY'RE GROWING

John Ioannidis is a physician-scientist, the director of the Stanford Prevention Research Center and co-director of the Meta-Research Innovation Center (METRIC). His 2005 paper, "Why Most Published Research Findings Are False" (Ioannidis, 2005) is the most downloaded technical paper from the journal PLoS Medicine. It is foundational to metascience, the use of scientific methods and to study science itself.

Ioannidis wrote that "a research finding is less likely to be true when the studies conducted in a field are smaller; when effect sizes are smaller; when there are a greater number and lesser preselection of tested relationship; where there is greater flexibility in designs, definitions, outcomes, and analytical modes; when there is greater financial and other interest and prejudice; and when more teams are involved in a scientific field in chase of statistical significance."

Most of those characteristics apply to the meta-analyses used by ACC/AHA Task Force on Practice Guidelines in their document "Guideline on the Assessment of Cardiovascular Risk" (Gogg, 2014).

The first CIMT meta-analysis was done by Pierluigi Costanzo and others, published in JACC (Journal of the American College of Cardiology) on December 2010 (Costanzo, 2010). This meta-analysis attempted to isolate and derive meaning from a series of studies which reviewed the relationship between CIMT and cardiovascular events.

"Using MEDLINE and Cochrane databases, randomized clinical trials up to 2009 using carotid IMT were analyzed. "A weighted random-effects meta-regression analysis was performed to test the relationship between mean and maximum IMT changes and outcomes (analogous to what is used to state arterial age). The influence of baseline patients' characteristics, cardiovascular risk profile, IMT at baseline, follow-up, and quality of trials was also explored. Overall estimates of effect were calculated with a fixed-effects model, random-effects model, or Peto method." (Costanzo, 2010)

"Results: Forty-one trials enrolling 18,307 participants were included. Despite significant reduction in CHD, CBV events, and all-cause death induced by active treatments (for CHD events, odds ratio (OR): 0.82...; for CBV events, OR: 0.71,...; and for all-cause death, OR: 0.71), there was no significant relationship between IMT regression and CHD events..., CBV events..., and all-cause death..." (Costanzo 2010)

"Conclusions: Regression or slowed progression of carotid IMT, induced by cardiovascular drug therapies, do not reflect a reduction in cardiovascular events." (Costanzo 2010)

In short, the meta-analysis conducted by this group did not demonstrate a relationship between lowering CIMT and lowered event rates. In other words, their study attempts to show that even if you change your CIMT, you do not necessarily decrease the risk of heart attacks and strokes.

Of course, this is counter to a wealth of pre-existing science studies (over 14,000), which were done using CIMT as a surrogate outcome, which showed the opposite. Why then does this meta-analysis differ in its apparent conclusion?

It is a fair question, and it gets to the very heart of the problem demonstrated in many meta-analyses.

We are not the only ones critical of the Costanzo article, or the standards committee's reliance on it. The following quote are from an editorial by James Stein, a cardiologist in Madison, Wisconsin, and an expert on CIMT responded to the article as a representative of the American College of Cardiology Foundation. (Stein, 2011)

"Costanzo et al. concluded that slowed the progression of… CIMT with drug therapies does not predict reduced cardiovascular disease (CVD) risk. Unfortunately, their analytical technique, meta-regression, is not suitable for evaluating this relationship. The limitations of meta-regression are well-known. Major pitfalls of their study including the following:" (Stein, 2011)

"1. CIMT is not a standardized technology. Their meta-regression included studies with different imaging and measurement techniques. By grouping them, the authors created a null bias. Furthermore, some laboratories have highly reproducible techniques and excellent quality assurance procedures. Those laboratories have reliably reported strong relationships between changes in CVD risk factors, changes in CIMT, and CVD risk. But some laboratories have poor measurement accuracy and reproducibility. Because the meta-regression lumped widely differing methodologies together, it is no surprise that they did not find a relationship among all the noise from the individual trials. Adjusting for the year of the study, the authors' proposed solution does not address this problem." (Stein, 2011)

"2. Short follow-up duration. CIMT progression studies are experiments that evaluate one biological effect of an intervention—change in carotid atherosclerosis burden (or more precisely, change in wall thickness, a measure of arterial injury). CIMT progression studies are performed to obtain information about the effect of an intervention on the arterial wall in a shorter time period than usually is needed to observe differences in CVD event rates… short-term events are more related to inflammation and thrombosis than atherosclerosis burden. Proponents of CIMT imaging as a research tool do not claim that CIMT changes perfectly reflect CVD risk, especially in the short term. Their analysis attacks a red herring and faults a technique for not predicting events that are not mediated by what it measures. Indeed, the Cholesterol Lowering Atherosclerosis Study showed a significant relationship between CIMT changes and lipid treatment after 2 years, but the relationships between changes in lipids, CIMT, and CVD events took many more years to be identified. The studies analyzed by Costanzo et al. were, for the most part, only 1 to 2 years in duration." (Stein, 2011)

"3. The meta-regression was performed on summary data, not data from individual study participants, and there were a lot of missing data—especially important considerations given the small number of CVD events they analyzed relative to the large number of covariates and studies in their models." (Stein, 2011). "No surrogate is perfect, but the vast majority of interventions that reduce CIMT progression also reduce CVD events. Exceptions include small, poorly conducted studies or interventions where the beneficial effect on CIMT was observed in different individuals than those with increased CVD risk (i.e., hormone replacement therapy). The limitations of meta-regression, short follow-up duration, and data limitations explain why the authors did not observe a relationship between CIMT changes and CVD events. It is noteworthy that another analysis that focused on high-quality CIMT studies of statins came to a different conclusion." (Stein, 2011) "

AMERICAN COLLEGE OF CARDIOLOGY

So, what Dr. Stein points out is that there are several problems in the way these researchers conducted their review.

First, they included many poor-quality studies in their analysis. Many of these studies were conducted by labs that had no prior CIMT experience. Would you include studies of surgery done by surgical teams with no previous experience?

The studies used different protocols (when they used a protocol at all). We have already discussed the importance a protocol makes with regards to reproducibility, sensitivity, and specificity. At best, this meta-analysis compared "apples and oranges."

In any study report, the goal is to write the experiment such that others could replicate it. The results obtained would then be obtained presumably by anyone else repeating the experiment. Yet many of the studies included in the analysis by the standards committees had no data available on processes or reliability. The committees included studies conducted by laboratories with no data on reproducibility and no published data on their quality metrics. There simply is no comparison.

The final point is that the study time was too short. Heart disease trials typically take 3 to 5 years and thousands of patients. Otherwise, there is just not enough statistical power to reliably demonstrate a difference between studied groups. This meta-analysis only looked at 1 to 2 years of data. There were not that many events in that time window. This also means that the reduction of events in the shortened time window was simply not observed. This is called an underpowered study. This underpowered study problem happened on not one, but two separate meta-analyses used by the standards committee to rule on whether to include recommending CIMT for routine use or not.

We are hopeful this will provide you with the additional insight needed to understand better the meta-analysis addressed above. It is important to note that as of this book's publication, there are over 14,000 peer-reviewed publications that have looked at CIMT technology. The FDA has allowed pharmaceutical companies, which manufacture drugs for the treatment of cardiovascular diseases, to use CIMT as a surrogate endpoint when testing their drugs for the past 30 years.

IMT does not measure a risk factor for CV disease. It directly measures and quantifies the amount of CV disease by measuring inflammation and plaque. These decisions by the medical standards committees have resulted in under-utilization of CIMT and over-reliance on Stress Tests and other less predictive technologies.

CIMT has proven utility in terms of sensitivity, specificity, reproducibility, and its unique ability to be used to monitor the efficacy of an intervention.

OTHERS HAVE QUESTIONED THE STRESS TEST: THE SHAPE STANDARDS

This book is not the first criticism of Stress Tests. Others have formed their own standards committees. An "international group of experts" formed a "task force" in 2006 "to address a major shortcoming in existing guidelines in the primary prevention of (CV disease)". Their findings were "based on the observation that most heart attacks and strokes occur in people who are not classified as high risk by the traditional risk factor-based approach recommended in the United States (Framingham Risk Score) and Europe (SCORE). " Consequently, the Screening for Heart Attack Prevention and Education (SHAPE) Task Force, began proposing its own guidelines (Naghavi, 2006).

"Unfortunately, these guidelines (from alternate standard's committees) provide inadequate warning to asymptomatic individuals with subclinical atherosclerosis who are unaware of their high-risk status and are not aggressively treated by their physicians who follow the existing recommendations. Consequently, most of these asymptomatic individuals, who are vulnerable to a near-future heart attack, are not offered the benefit of existing prophylactic therapies. Unlike decades ago, when screening for risk factors of A-CVD was the only available risk stratification method in primary prevention, today, noninvasive detection of atherosclerosis is feasible and widely available. It provides a direct and individualized method for risk assessment. A large body of evidence has been compiled in recent years showing the superior prognostic value of detecting atherosclerosis rather than risk factors of atherosclerosis. The First SHAPE Guideline calls for noninvasive screening of all asymptomatic men 45 to 75 years old and asymptomatic women 55 to 75 years old (except those defined as very low risk) to detect and treat individuals with subclinical atherosclerosis. The intensity of treatment should correlate with the severity of the disease. Among existing tools for detection of subclinical atherosclerosis, the SHAPE Task Force has created the SHAPE Flow Chart based on the following 2 noninvasive imaging techniques: coronary artery calcium scoring using computed tomography and cartotid intima media thickness (CIMT) and plaque using B-mode ultrasonography."

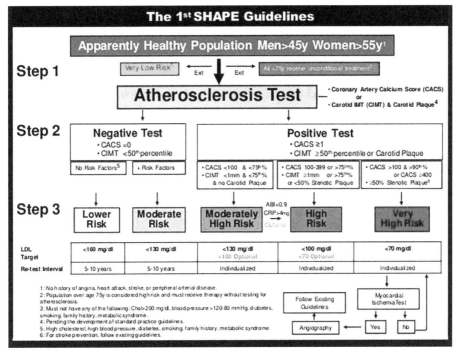

Source: (Naghavi, 2006)

As can be seen in the guideline document above, the SHAPE guideline also encouraged earlier and more frequent use of the non-invasive screening tests (Coronary Calcium Score and CIMT).

WHAT HAPPENED TO THE SHAPE TASK FORCE?

There is a small YouTube channel (shapesociety) with 157 subscribers. The founder of the SHAPE task force, Dr. Morteza Naghavi of Houston, heads up the (shapesociety) YouTube channel, a group of "centers of excellence", and a couple of start-ups involved in CV prevention screening and treatment (Endothelix and DTM endothelial function testing). This movement certainly does not appear to be on a path to unseat stress testing, the catheter lab, and stents any time soon.

The SHAPE task force and standards have a lot going for them. They may have been before their time. As mentioned, they were formed and seemed to fade away before:

Todd C Eldredge PHD, MPH, MBA | 159 | Ford Brewer, MD, MPH

- The ISCHEMIA trial showed that bypass grafts don't prevent heart attacks (Herman 2019);
- The COURAGE & other trials showed that stents don't prevent heart attacks (Boden 2007);
- ORBITA indicated that stents might not even help angina (Al-Lamee 2018);
- The USPSTF acknowledged improvement in risk assessment using "nontraditional" risk factors (USPSTF 2018);
- The ACC/AHA endorsed focusing on "the simple 7" (Turco, 2018);
- The ABIM Foundation formed Choosing Wisely to discourage overuse of interventions like stress tests, angiograms and stent (ChoosingWisely.org);
- Blaha and others from Johns Hopkins encouraged addition of the "nontraditional" risk factors (Kolata 2013).

The list goes on.

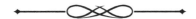

PATIENT STORIES, RISK FACTORS, TESTS & MORE SCIENCE

REVERSING INFLAMMATION AND PLAQUE – "MY CARDIOLOGIST SAYS THAT'S IMPOSSIBLE"

Most patients and doctors think CV disease cannot be reversed. A quick Google scholar search for keywords like "artery plaque reversal" produces over 6 million science citations on those keywords alone. Plenty of medical scientists have demonstrated plaque reversal using several methods, including IMT studies, calcium scans, and even autopsies.

Thomas Lee, MD, Editor-in-Chief of the Harvard Health Letter, covered this issue first in January 2009 and again in March 2019. He focused on significant weight loss as a method to reverse inflammation in the arterial wall. His first response was, "If you have the gumption to make major changes to your lifestyle, you can, indeed, reverse coronary artery disease". He described the loss of plaque in autopsies of WW2 victims who died from starvation. He mentioned Dean Ornish's "reversal diet". Lee also described the impact of statins. "Studies… with statins… have yielded mixed results… they still reduce rates of heart attack and stroke. They do this by decreasing the amount of fluid fat inside the plaque, by stabilizing the covering over it, and by calming inflammation. Dryer plaques with tougher, more fibrous caps are less likely to break open and cause heart attacks". (Harvard University, 2006).

Starving to decrease CV disease does not sound like an appealing option. But the loss of 30 pounds of fat is a different issue. We see many patients that have lost 30 pounds or more (recently more than one had lost over 150 pounds). These weight loss experiences still do not reliably reverse plaque. If you go back to the original images of inflammation, you see an inflammatory soup of cells, enzymes, chemicals, and cellular trash. Fibrous tissue (scarring) and calcium can replace that inflammatory soup. That calcified plaque is shrunken in volume from the previous soft plaque. It is also stable. (Honda 2004)

THE MOST COMMON METHOD OF WEIGHT LOSS

The pattern in motivated patients tends to be the same. James West & Gene Lovell used this technique. Dozens of other patients have said the same. First, they go low carb which tends to decrease hunger. Second, they narrow their eating window. The most common term used for this approach to weight loss is intermittent fasting. Valter Longo and Satchin Panda would call it time-restricted feeding (Longo, 2016).

In most cases, we call it skipping breakfast. Some use OMAD (One Meal a Day). Others have used ProLon, Longo's FMD (Fasting Mimicking Diet). A few have even added prolonged fasting to their menu. The biomedical changes demonstrated in research on prolonged fasting make it easy to recommend it as a vehicle to reverse metabolic syndrome and to affect changes in the arterial wall. Recent science indicates it improves health even without weight loss.

WEIGHT LOSS DOESN'T ALWAYS PREVENT HEART ATTACKS

Chuck, the engineer in Ford's YouTube channel video "Wild Ride," lost 50 pounds on a vegan diet. Based on advice from a well-known plant-based doctor, he continued to focus on decreasing fats and oils, even those from plants (like nuts). After losing 50 pounds, Chuck had a heart attack. He began watching the channel and realized he might have insulin resistance. You will also hear Insulin Resistance called Prediabetes or Metabolic Syndrome. It is the primary cause of CV inflammation and, therefore, plaque. IR is far more common than has been recognized. The CDC estimates there are over 80 million Americans with this condition. 90% of them do not know it. These estimates are conservative. The CDC based them on criteria that are known to have high false-negative rates (fasting glucose and HgA1c) (CDC, July 18, 2017). As mentioned elsewhere, UCLA estimates are that over half the adult population are insulin resistant (Babey SH, 2016).

THE SCOPE OF THIS BOOK IS PLAQUE MEASUREMENT, NOT LIFESTYLE CHANGES

Further details behind the management of CV risk are beyond the scope of this book; our purpose is to improve plaque screening and measurement. In the rest of this chapter, we will provide stories demonstrating plaque reversal.

FORD' PLAQUE REVERSAL STORY

"At age 56, I had my first CIMT. I had recently retired from a stressful corporate job. But in many ways, I found retirement even more stressful.

"Some friends in the preventive medicine space asked my opinion of Brad Bale and Amy Doneen's book 'Beat the Heart Attack Gene'. I read the book several times and attended one of Brad and Amy's seminars. A vendor was providing CIMT to attendees. I visited and had my CIMT exam completed. We give that story in the CIMT section of this book.

" Most situations of plaque reversal involve weight loss or the initiation of statins in people with young plaque. All three applied to my story.

"Our practice at PrevMed included CIMTs, so I got my own CIMT every few months. You could see a linear progression of improvement. How much of this effect was due to weight loss vs. the statins vs. other things? I will never know. Still, I do know that my inflammation shrunk, and my arterial health improved."

FORD'S CIMTS DEMONSTRATING INFLAMMATION REVERSAL

CardioRisk™ Scan Patient Results

Patient Name: BREWER, FORD
Gender: M
Date of Exam: 9/17/2016
Date of Birth: 6/27/1957
Referring Provider: BALE DONEEN CONFERENCE

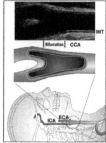

| Patient Age | 59 | Patient IMT | 0.78 mm |
| Arterial Age | 63 | Normal IMT | < .50 mm |

CV Event Risk   All measurements in mm

Test Criteria:	Normal	Moderate	High	Last Visit (2015)*	Alert Value*
Early Event Risk⁺⁺	1.5			1.5	2
Average CCA Mean IMT	0.67			0.74	0.73
Average CCA Max Region	0.71			0.81	0.75
Plaque Burden**			1.5	1.5	

Comments: The following values are the largest intima-media thickness (IMT) measurements found in each carotid artery segment. Any measurement equal to or 1.3mm is defined as 'plaque' and is characterized as being: S = Soft; H = Heterogeneous; or E = Echogenic (includes mineral deposits like calcium). All measurements are in millimeters.

Right CCA .8; Bulb 1.5 H; Internal Carotid .7
Left CCA .8; Bulb .8; Internal Carotid .7
Doppler was used bilaterally.

	Exam Date	Age at Exam	Arterial Age	CIMT	Percentile
🤍	Nov 2019	62	55	0.69	38th
🤍	Apr 2018	60	53	0.68	37th
🤍	Sep 2016	59	52	0.67	37th
🤍	Oct 2015	58	59	0.74	54th
❤️	Feb 2015	57	73	0.88	84th

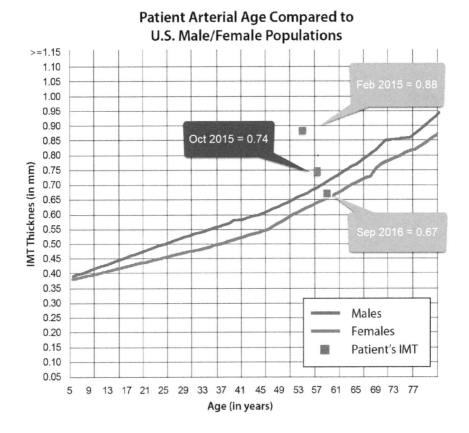

JOHN'S STORY

John's background and weight loss/progress

John had been studying health and wellness for years. He ran a sophisticated health discussion forum. John had completed several Coronary Calcium Scores. Many advised him against this for two reasons. One, Coronary Calcium Scores are not usually discrete enough to detect progression. Two, many people worry about the radiation from Coronary Calcium Scores. (John's decision was well-informed. We cover this in the previous sections on radiation and Coronary Calcium Scores.)

John was frustrated that he had no explanation for the steady climb in his Coronary Calcium Score. After watching our channel, he rechecked his sugars. His doctor checked them routinely and his numbers were good, or so he thought. He humored Dr. Brewer in his request to get an OGTT. You will recall that this is the test where the patient's blood is drawn and tested for glucose. Then we challenge the patient's pancreas by having the patient drink a measured dose of glucose – a sugary drink. Blood is subsequently drawn and measured at the 1hr, 2hr intervals, and sometimes 3 hours following the administration of this substance.

The results are below.

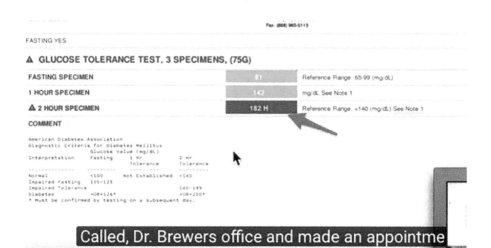

Source: Ford Brewer's YouTube Channel

John's blood sugar peaked at 184 on the OGTT. He agreed to get a Kraft insulin survey (a Kraft insulin survey or Prediabetes Profile is a timed test that measures the insulin response to a glucose challenge and returns to baseline over 4 hours. The insulin survey shows patterns of insulin response rather than a strict cut-off point for glucose). John's Kraft study demonstrated what Kraft calls a "type 2 response," a delayed insulin peak.

As mentioned before, undiagnosed insulin resistance is the primary driver of arterial disease. That makes it the cause of most chronic disease, death, and disability. Also as mentioned earlier, this book will not go into a detailed explanation of this topic – we will leave that for other books. Joseph Kraft's book "The Diabetes Epidemic and You" is a good read for those interested. It demonstrates the growing frequency of the problem with aging. (Kraft 2009)

"THOSE TESTS ARE RIGGED TO FAIL"

As John shared in his videos, his primary care doc said he "didn't know what to do with these test results," since they were "rigged to fail". There are 100 grams of sugar in a Kraft insulin survey. According to the Coca-Cola website, that is less than the amount of sugar in 32 ounces of Coke, or a large Coke at McDonald's. (www.cocacolaproductfacts.com/en/faq/sugar/how-much-sugar-in-coke/)

As John shared in another video, his ophthalmologist told him there were diabetic changes in his eyes. That was further evidence he had landed on the right problem.

Maybe John's doctor did not know what to do with the test results, but John did. He cut his carbs, lost 40 pounds, and got his daily blood sugars down. Even directly following a meal, his blood sugars did not go over 100 anymore. His blood pressure dropped. He had to stop most of his blood pressure medications.

John decided to seek verification on his progress by doing another Coronary Calcium Score. As you can see from the title of the video, John's Coronary Calcium Score dropped by 59%. I have only seen a couple of significant drops in Coronary Calcium Score previously. While some of this change could be attributed to different techniques and equipment – it would be hard to attribute this much of a change to protocol or error in the method. You can find the video here: *https://youtu.be/ysifMKWKZLY*.

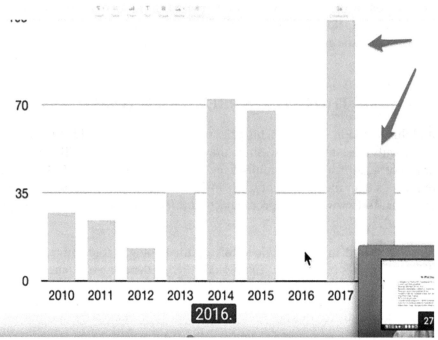

Source: Ford Brewer's YouTube Channel https://youtu.be/ysifMKWKZLY

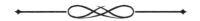

PATIENT STORIES

ANNA'S STORY - A FAMILY WITH Lp(a), AND INSULIN RESISTANCE

Anna was a 56-year-old Mexican American. She told us her family had significant heart attack risk, even for a Hispanic American. Her father, both brothers and other family members had heart attacks in their 50s. She was a biomedical professional. The family was looking for her to help solve this problem. She had reviewed cholesterol values in the family. They seemed to be fine.

Anna was attending one of our events, hoping to find clues. She was also hoping she could avoid the problem herself. Unfortunately, her CIMT indicated her arterial age was ten years older than her chronological age (64 vs. 54). As she suspected, cholesterol was not the problem. Her LDL, for example, was 71. During our discussions following the first day's meeting, she disclosed that she thought she had discovered the problem.

Anna's Lp(a) was 281. Lp(a) is a common genetic variant of LDL. When some people make a high amount of Lp(a) variant, their risk increases (Wilde 2003). The medical community continues to debate over lab cut points and whether treatments (such as niacin) work. Most standards committees still do not recommend screening for this risk factor. Failure to screen for a risk factor known to be present in at least 20% of the population is another questionable decision on the part of standards committees such as the ACC/AHA. That debate has increased significantly since The Biggest Loser star Bob Harper stated that Lp(a) caused his heart attack (Arnett, 2019) (Scheel, 2019).

Elevated Lp(a) certainly is a risk factor. Many of the patients we see have elevated Lp(a). They often do not have problems until other critical risk factors enter the picture. Prediabetes is the most common risk factor that presents itself to the mix.

Anna had risk factors for prediabetes. Although few would describe her as overweight, her BMI (in the high 20s) and fat mass were too high. Body fat used to be considered inert storage, now it is known to be an endocrine tissue. Body fat secretes hormones that cause insulin resistance and CV inflammation. Her OGTT (see Glossary) results were unusually good for a 54-year-old woman with 64-year-old arteries.

At the time her OGTT was completed, the lab did not offer insulin values for all three blood samples of the OGTT. Now the lab has added insulin values, making this similar to a Kraft Insulin Survey (see Glossary).

Anna had not heard of Lp(a) before coming to our event. She started on niacin and successfully lowered her Lp(a). That was fortunate. Upon leaving the program, she reported feeling immense relief. It was now possible to help save her family as well as herself.

JIM'S STORY

Many think that staying thin assures decreased CV risk. That is not always true. Low weight, however, is often a sign of reduced muscle mass, especially as we age beyond our mid-60s. Sarcopenia ("Sarco" means muscle, and "penia" means loss) is one of the most significant risk factors for adults over 65. Increased fat mass is one of the most common risk factors, especially in the aging population. Our next story is about another thin individual that still developed significant risk at an early age.

Jim was tall and thin. At 6 feet, 7 inches, and 175 pounds, his BMI was only 20.5. Jim was muscular with very little body fat. By the age of 53, however, he had already had two stents. What was causing this problem? Did he have a genetic variation of cholesterol (like FH - Familial Hypercholesterolemia)? Or was this problem associated with an earlier case of diabetes? Was it attributable to an undiagnosed inflammatory disease like rheumatoid arthritis? Was there a history of smoking in his background resulting in plaque formation?

Previous LDL cholesterol values had been typical. With normal CIMT, LDL, and very little fat mass, Jim's case started as a puzzle. Pre-stent angiograms showed plaque. Because of Jim's height and low BMI, Marfan's syndrome was considered.

Marfan's syndrome was first described by the French pediatrician Antoine Marfan in 1896. Patients with Marfan's syndrome are usually thin and often tall. They can also have other conditions such as abnormal joint mobility. Marfan's syndrome can result in early death, often while patients are in their 30s. Premature death from Marfan's is quite different from a heart attack. In Marfan's, the aorta can split and leak.

Jim's doctors had considered Marfan's several years before and had ruled it out. However, it was still possible that Jim had one of the Marfanoid syndromes, such as Stickler's syndrome. Stickler's syndrome is the most common connective tissue disorder in Europe and the US. Jim's mother had a history suggestive of Stickler's; she had a retinal detachment and knee replacement (Verma, 2008).

Then Jim's lab values returned. Jim's Lp(a) was over 300. He started niacin. Less than four months later, his Lp(a) dropped to just over 200. He has been on statins since before his first stent. Statins do not help Lp(a); they can increase it (Tsimikas, 2019). Jim is relieved to find a problem he can manage. He has gone back to an old habit - exercising.

A NEW FUTURE FOR PEOPLE WITH Lp(a)

There is new hope for people with elevated Lp(a). In early January of 2020, the New England Journal published the first big clinical trial of a new class of drugs (antisense drugs) for Lp(a). (Tsimikas 2019). Many Lp(a) patients want to join further studies. Others want these new antisense drugs now. That is understandable, but it will take time to understand the indications and risks of these drugs. They will also likely be expensive until competition increases in this specific drug space. The current generation will still have challenges as we work through these issues. There's little question as to whether Lp(a) will be an issue for the next generation.

ANGIE'S STORY

Angie is the 50-year-old wife of a physician. Both she and the physician are Ford's patients. She expected to have no CV problems. Her CIMT came back, showing 60-year-old arteries. Up until her initial visit, Angie focused on her Hashimoto's disease and GI (gastrointestinal) symptoms. She was not aware that she had elevated CV risk. The same problem causing her Hashimoto's and GI symptoms might have increased her CV risk.

Systemic inflammation, often seen with Hashimoto's disease, is often attributable to a common genetic variation called haptoglobin 2. Dr. Alessio Fasano originally described Haptoglobin 2 as the cause of leaky gut. Nobody believed him, at least at first. Now things have changed.

Fasano and others have shown that Haptoglobin 2, and its precursor (zonulin) cause multiple inflammatory diseases ranging from CV disease to leaky gut, to Hashimoto's. They have demonstrated the genetic and amino acid sequence of Haptoglobin 2 and zonulin (Fasano, 2005).

People like Angie are now finding surprising causes for their thyroid disease as well as their CV inflammation. Dr. Fasano is now the head of an extensive zonulin research program at Harvard and the chief of Pediatric Gastroenterology at Mass General.

Angie also had prediabetes. Her BMI was 29 and her fasting glucose was over 100. She was not surprised to find that weight loss was going to be a significant part of her journey back to health.

Armed with better data, Angie was motivated to work more diligently on her lifestyle which had an immediate effect on her BMI and her fasting glucose. She was able to get her BMI down to 23 and her fasting glucose down to 83. Her CIMT rewarded her efforts and showed a slight decrease in the arterial wall inflammation bringing her arterial age back below 50. Perhaps most importantly, Angie feels motivated to continue to work on her BMI and completely move out of the pre-diabetes risk group. This has long-term positive ramifications not just in terms of her health and potential diabetes but also in terms of significantly reduced risk of heart attack or stroke – but the most important benefit is how she feels. Angie reports increased energy and zest for life and it never hurts to be happy at what one sees when they look at the mirror.

BAILEY'S STORY - IF, CR, TRF, AND OTHER ACRONYMS

Bailey is a hygienist. She was 40 years old, but her CIMT showed she had arteries that were equivalent to those of a 57-year-old. Her BMI was 29. Bailey's blood work indicated she was prediabetic. Weight loss had to be a top priority. It had already been an area of concern and focus. She had tried unsuccessfully to lose weight to look better. She did not realize it was adversely impacting her heart health.

A year later, after having lost 20 pounds, she felt great, and she looked great too. She admits that the CIMT was the catalytic event; it motivated her to finally lose the weight. After she started with us, she found better ways to lose weight. First, she went on a low carb diet. Dropping the amount of carbs stopped her recurring hunger. David Ludwig, an endocrinologist and dietary researcher at Harvard, wrote a book on carbohydrates and weight. The title of his book, "Always Hungry", tells a vital part of the story (Ludwig, 2016).

After a month of eating fewer carbs, she added what she calls "intermittent fasting" (IF). Yes, she also started skipping breakfast. John's story in the previous chapter demonstrates the value of IF. We also introduced other forms of IF and TRF (Time-Restricted Feeding). Science has shown for over 30 years that dietary Caloric Restriction (CR) dramatically improves the lifespan of many species (Weindruch, 1997). Early studies indicated that decreased oxidation was the key (Sohal, 1996). But studies since then have indicated that the benefits from intermittent fasting are not merely the results of reduced free-radical production or weight loss (Longo V. M., 2014) (Longo V. P., 2016) (DiFrancesco, 2018).

It appears that intermittent fasting elicits adaptive cellular responses that improve glucose regulation, increase stress resistance, and suppress inflammation. During a fast, cells activate pathways that enhance natural defenses against oxidative and metabolic stress and those that remove or repair damaged molecules. During feeding periods, cells engage in growth and plasticity (DeCabo, 2019).

Most people consume three meals daily plus snacks in an eating window lasting from early morning to late evening, so they never give their bodies a chance to switch into the fat-burning burning mode. Metabolic switching is required to decrease CV inflammation and other things that go with aging (Longo V. P., 2016).

We suggested that Bailey add prolonged water fasts (two days or more), to emphasize the beneficial changes in metabolism. The prolonged water fasts are not a popular option, but they can be powerful. Valter Longo created a five-day diet designed to make fasting easier. The goal is to trick the body into thinking it is fasting. He has demonstrated positive effects, including reversal of CV inflammation and insulin resistance. The goal is to reverse decades of epigenetics (programming of our DNA's "librarian") to make it easier to find the genes and make the proteins needed to burn fat and recycled cellular components (Longo V. P., 2016).

Bailey's subsequent CIMT showed that the inflammation in her arterial wall had been arrested and that the intermittent fasting and prolonged water fasts had affected the desired changes. This means that Bailey's long-term risk of heart attack and stroke have been significantly reduced.

AMIT'S STORY

Amit was a 39-year-old Indian American businessman whose CIMT results showed he had 54-year-old equivalent arteries. He worked in finance and IT. His BMI was 28. He was clearly "headed down that diabetic highway". Following his CIMT exam which provided him with significant motivation to improve his health he began a strict health regimen. After getting started with his health protection plan or regimen, he lost 30 pounds. He plans to lose at least 5 more. His OGTT and HbA1c have improved as has his CIMT. Like many of us, his glucose metabolism is extremely sensitive to his weight and fat mass. If he regains that 30 pounds of fat mass, he will likely see his glucose metabolism, his arterial and general health and wellness decline again.

JAKE'S STORY - FH VS. LEAN MASS HYPER RESPONDER

"I got my cholesterol tested when I was 19 or 20 years old. Even at that age, I had high cholesterol. I have a great deal of heart disease on both sides of my family. My dad recently had a triple bypass. He's always had trouble controlling his cholesterol … he's like me, thin and athletic. I'm young, 40 with 2 kids. I researched this a lot. I couldn't get my LDL below 200… I worked out, I watched my diet, I got a Coronary Calcium Score. It freaked me out. At age 39, I had a positive Coronary Calcium Score. No longer did I just have a risk of disease, I had a disease. I'm very disciplined. I read Ivor Cummins' (low carb diet) book (Cummins, 2018). I fully embraced it, but when I got tested, my total cholesterol was 460. My LDL was 379, it was ridiculous. That's when I started watching (Ford's) YouTube channel. I needed someone that understood both sides of it. I needed to rule out insulin resistance. I needed a balanced approach. I wasn't going to do this entirely with lifestyle. Now I've got numbers that are beyond my wildest dreams. It's been a huge process. I've got Familial Hypercholesterolemia along with - I'm a lean mass hyper responder. I don't do keto anymore, but I do have a low carb diet." (Video from the YouTube channel https://www.youtube.com/watch?v=tcdpkXKefzE)

Dave Feldman is another engineer on the internet who is focusing on cardiovascular disease. (https://cholesterolcode.com/about/). He focuses on what he calls Lean Mass Hyper Responder. He describes people that get an increase in cholesterol when they cut carbs. It is nothing new to see cholesterol rising in response to low carb diets, but there are now new ways of seeing it. There are over 2000 genetic variations of FH, or Familial Hypercholesterolemia. Some of those people with FH can turn out to be Lean Mass Hyper Responders.

DAVID'S STORY

David is a 62-year-old with significant insulin resistance, bordering on full diabetes. He had a stroke 2 years ago. His docs always told him everything was fine. They did not know what caused the TIA. As recently as 2 months ago, they told him his blood sugars were fine. One and two hours after drinking the 75-gram challenge of glucose, his blood sugars were 198 and 175 – which is too high, and borderline diabetic. His corresponding insulin values were 121 and 135. His response was, "I've never had a stress test, but I'm getting a CIMT. I watch your channel". David had a soft plaque on his CIMT exam, these are extremely dangerous because they can easily rupture or erode. He is now extremely motivated and moving quickly on his campaign to lose fat mass.

Given our extensive history with this type of patient, we can anticipate the inflammation in David's arteries to attenuate and the soft plaque will collect calcium and collagen and become completely hardened over time if he will continue to drop his blood sugar and insulin production.

JEFF'S STRESS TEST - EXECUTIVE EXAMS AND THE WORRIED WELL

Jeff's story illustrates why stress tests, cardiologists and university faculty may not be the best options for the evaluation of CV risk and the risk of heart attack or stroke.

Some people think of executive exam programs as inappropriate perks for wealthy executives. However, the human resources head at these companies see their executives as high-value corporate assets. They are only looking for ways to protect these assets. Corporations see these executive examination programs as an investment, a type of insurance against the loss of leadership talent. Human resource leaders have included stress tests in their executive exam programs for decades. Many Human resource directors are informed enough to know that stress tests are inadequate insurance against heart attacks, but they do not know about a better solution. They certainly do not want to lose an executive to a heart attack on their watch without at least taking the old school "protective" measures (e.g. stress tests). Also, many executives are well informed and understand that an annual stress test does almost nothing to evaluate their real risk of having a heart attack or stroke. Those participating in these programs are often in the "worried well" category.

One of these was an executive named Jeff, a 40-year-old ultramarathon runner. He was a little worried about some vague symptoms he had while running for a couple of weeks. Unlike many of us, he at least brought these symptoms to his physician's attention. Despite his symptoms, Jeff declined inflammation testing, IR (insulin resistance) testing, and CIMT.

Instead, he went to a well-known cardiologist at a nearby academic medical center who did a Nuclear Stress Test. Jeff returned confident that a heart attack was only remotely possible. He was able to get to a high level of exertion on the treadmill. What ultramarathoner would not? Jeff did not know the Tim Russert story. His cardiologist knew little about CV inflammation. Most cardiologists do not know much about arterial inflammation. Jeff did not know what to do about it. He also probably knew a little about the dangers and ubiquity of prediabetes. Again, most cardiologists know that, but most do not know what to do about it.

OUR LAST STORY: GERRY'S STROKE AND STEM CELL THERAPY

Gerry was a 66-year-old man when we first met four years ago. He was exhausted all the time. On a good day, he could go up a flight or two of stairs. Most days, he could not. He also drags his left leg as a result of the stroke he experienced a year earlier.

Fatigue is common in over half of all stroke patients. Post-stroke fatigue interferes with everyday life. It bothered Gerry's family more than seeing him drag his left leg. They lived in Texas, where Gerry had a mid-level executive position in a local business. Gerry's passion had always been his small cattle ranch. He had been able to maintain profitability for many years when others could not. He kept his debt low and had access to favorable buyers and graze lots. One of his strengths was that he needed fewer employees. He was the energizer bunny of small ranchers.

While he worked at the company to provide financial security for his family, he worked at the ranch for fun, whenever he could. After the stroke, however, that all stopped. He tells strangers that his case is still a good fortune—that the stroke did not put him in a wheelchair, but his family knew the rest of the story. The stroke took his beloved ranch away, and that took away Gerry's reason for living.

Gerry was tough; this was not his first rodeo with fatigue. As an active rancher, working his ranch during the off-hours of a busy corporate job, he routinely dealt with fatigue. There were three keys to his ability to cope with his rigorous schedule: staying in good shape, pushing through fatigue, and getting naps. These things had always worked for him.

After the stroke, though, this was no longer the case. Gerry is a fighter. He pushed himself for the entire year following his stroke, resorting to naps and weight loss to improve his stamina, but things did not improve. The family wanted help for him. Unfortunately, this type of morbid (or disease-related) fatigue happens in about 2/3 of all stroke patients. The cause is not well-understood, but it can be devastating. While it usually lasts six months or less, it can last for years.

His family called to talk about stem cell treatment. They read about stem cell treatment patients having a total cure and being completely free from their post-stroke fatigue and other symptoms. Was this real or were these just isolated stories. Could it be something worse? Stories promoted by today's version of yesterday's snake-oil salesmen. Some remarkable cures, like a study conducted at Stanford, lent credibility to the stem cell treatments.

We contacted a neurosurgeon friend involved in stem cell treatment for strokes. He offered the family a couple of options. Improvement with stem cell therapy was remote. Still, the family wanted to try them. The family recently returned from Mexico, their third offshore experience with stem cell therapy providers. They were desperate.

Gerry had a simple problem with prediabetes, and he successfully dealt with it. After finding out about his insulin resistance, Gerry lost the weight and got the carbs out of his diet. Before this, his glucose ranged from over 170 to just below 120. Over time, his inflammation and plaque stabilized, and his health improved.

Unfortunately, it was too late as far as the damage from the stroke was concerned. Nothing, including stem cell therapy, could cure the long-term sequelae or lingering effects of Gerry's stroke. Had he known about his insulin resistance earlier, he could have prevented it.

It is essential to tell Gerry's story to emphasize the need for prevention. However, that is not the only purpose of this story. Another aim is to compare research between stem cell therapy and IMT. The scientific evidence for preventive testing via CIMT is far stronger than that for stem cell treatment. Why then was Gerry never screened with a CIMT, an OGTT, a Kraft insulin survey, or inflammation testing?

There is no comparison between the science behind CIMT and that of stem cell therapy. So why would Gerry's family deplete his life savings on unfounded treatments?

The reason is obvious: Gerry's life had been devastated by his stroke. You could blame his doctors. Neither he nor his family knew about the prediabetes. Doctors rarely willfully neglect or misinform their patients. The medical practice environment drives these errors.

Doctors leave training with an understanding of the importance of lifestyle to health but stop advising this due to repeated refusals by patients. Insurance companies decrease compensation, so doctors respond by spending less time with patients. Patients and insurance companies demand prescriptions and procedures, so that is what doctors provide.

Gerry had three negative stress tests before his stroke. The only difference between Gerry's story and Tim Russert's was the final landing place of the clot.

GERRY AND TIM RUSSERT HAD A PREVENTABLE, RECONGIZABLE DISEASE PROCESS

Why weren't the right tests and therapy done? CIMT, a Coronary Calcium Score, OGTT or insulin survey, and inflammation panel would have told a different story. Why weren't they done?

There is a big gap in healthcare today. That gap is costing US citizens billions of dollars. Far more importantly, it is robbing us of decades of healthy life. It is the single biggest reason why the incidence of heart attacks and strokes has only been reduced minimally over the past few decades. That gap is the failure to diagnose insulin resistance or prediabetes and other conditions known to cause CV disease, heart attacks and strokes. The CDC knows it and is beginning to publish statements to this effect. Most medical standards committees still seem too focused on procedures and medications to give much attention to this problem.

Physician's offices are still behind the changing standards. The primary tools used today in most physician's offices are cholesterol screening and blood pressure. Cholesterol screening is a 70-year-old technology, and blood pressure is 120 years old. These tests can still be useful, but they are not a replacement for what is needed.

Technology has improved and science has come a long way in 70 years, so we need to embrace the new technologies which have been demonstrated to be effective. As presented earlier, in a 10-year, 100,000 person-year study, IMT correctly identified 98.6% of those patients who went on to have a heart attack or stroke. (Belcaro, 2001)

IMT identified them successfully before they had their event (e.g. heart attack or stroke). That is a better 'catch rate' than a home pregnancy test. The obvious question is: Why is that newer technology not being used routinely in every primary care physician's office in the world? Indeed, physicians should be asking themselves what tool or tools they have in their toolbox that can compare with those kinds of results. Primary care physicians (as a group) treat symptoms and risk factors but not the disease.

While the standards committees play a critical role in this space, medical providers must use the array of evidence available to them in peer-reviewed literature to improve the diagnosis, assessment, and the treatment of the disease if we are to reduce the morbidity and mortality of this pernicious disease.

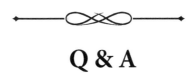

Q & A

Q: Wait a minute. I got one of those CIMTs already. It said I had no blockage of flow.

A: It sounds like you got a simple carotid ultrasound. That is a flow study. It is not a CIMT. Flow studies do not show plaque. Providers reading a carotid flow study just guess about the extent of plaque. Their recommendations are limited to carotid surgery. A carotid flow study is also called a Doppler or Duplex because it uses both B-Mode (brightness mode technology) and Doppler. A quality CIMT exam utilizes both B mode and Doppler as well. The difference is that the CIMT focusses on the arterial wall and measures the amount of inflammation and/or plaque whereas the Duplex or Doppler exam focuses on the velocity and direction of blood flow which requires blockage or a hemodynamic disturbance before showing "abnormal" on the report.

Q: How do they estimate "Arterial Age™?" Is that real? Is it like "real age"?

A: Arterial Age™ is a proprietary tool developed by CardioRisk which uses sophisticated statistical measures, including linear regression, to estimate a person's age equivalent when compared to large population studies which were conducted on studied populations. The Arterial Age™ is a coefficient of the Average CCA Mean IMT measurement which is derived from approximately 600 measurements taken from the arterial images which are taken during a CardioRisk exam. The Average CCA Mean IMT measurement by CardioRisk has been demonstrated to be accurate and reproducible in peer-reviewed, published data to an arithmetic difference of only 0.002mm (Riches, 2010). This makes the measurement extremely reliable and useful for tracking purposes.

These CIMT measurements were then organized by age to form a nomogram or normal CIMT distribution by age. Nomograms are graphs of average or normal values by age and gender from large epidemiological studies.

Yes, the data is real. It is important to understand, however, that the data upon which CardioRisk's Arterial Age™ is based excludes some of the highest risk population . . . those who died from the disease. As a result, the Arterial Age™ may understate risk, as those individuals who succumbed to the disease and were therefore excluded from the study, would have most likely had significant disease and certainly more disease than the remaining population. Arterial Age™ is better than the terms you have heard in the past, called "real age" or "vascular age". Arterial Age™ is a reliable Health Risk Appraisal.

Access outside of the US

Q: I live in Australia/Brazil/England/etc. How will I ever get the IMT? Here is a related comment/note: How do I access a valid CIMT? And how do I know if it's a good one?

A: CardioRisk offers its CIMT certification training program throughout the world. The certification training is completed when participants complete the double-blind, performance-based certification which is required by all those who seek certification. The double-blind, performance-based certification assures that the protocol is followed in a competent and reproducible manner and is certified by the International Society of Clinical Intima Media Ultrasonography (ISCIMU). The training classes have been completed all over the world. or can be completed by a single trip to their headquarters in Salt Lake City, UT. Dr. Eldredge has been teaching doctors and their clinical staff these techniques for decades. Having participated in parts of the training myself, I can attest to the fact that it was rigorous.

That experience actually gave me much more respect for CardioRisk's IMT quality and training programs. As a doc seeing patients, this is what I see: mostly patients (and docs) that did not understand the difference between CIMT and Doppler ultrasound. Then I see some that are labeled by the radiologist as CIMT.

However, these ultrasounds rarely have important data on them such as Mean Max or Average Mean CIMT. As we have discussed, I have a couple of reactions to these. First, it indicates that they do not know the science. The science indicates that Mean Max is a critical number.

Stress testing

Q: In the chapter on stress testing, you refer to the EKG. Is that the same as an ECG? Doesn't it stand for electrocardiogram? And if it does, why does the more popular term (EKG) contain a "K"?

Yes, the terms EKG and ECG are the same for these purposes. They do stand for electrocardiogram. The "K" comes from the German spelling of the word.

Here is what happened. The major time of development of this technique for tracking the heart signals was during the late 19th century (the late 1800s). In 1905, Dr. William Einthoven, a Dutch physiologist, recorded the first human electrocardiogram. He then transmitted this to his lab from the hospital (about a mile away). Dr. Einthoven was awarded the 1924 Nobel Prize for Medicine or Physiology for his work on the electrocardiogram.

That just provides a little history of this critical biomedical test. It does not tell the origin of the "K" here. Germany was the hotbed of the development in the science of medicine at that time (late 19th century). Dr. Einthoven was in the Netherlands and spoke German. The German term for ECG is "Elektro Kardio Gram" or EKG.

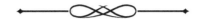

GLOSSARY OF TERMS

9P21 - 9P21 is also known as "the heart attack gene." 9P21 is a location on the 9th chromosome. It was initially associated with cancers, then heart attack, then diabetes. There are multiple specific points (SNPs) and numerous genetic variations leading to diabetes as well as weak artery walls. 9P21 is quite common.

ABI - Ankle Brachial Index - The ABI is a comparison of the ankle and arm blood pressures. If the ankle pressure is low compared to the arm, this implies vascular dysfunction of the arteries, and could be indicative of arterial plaque. This test is simple in concept but requires robust quality systems.

ABIM - American Board of Internal Medicine

ACC - American College of Cardiology

ACC/AHA Guidelines - The ACC/AHA Clinical practice guidelines were written by the American College of Cardiology/American Heart Association Task Force on Clinical Practice Guidelines. For purposes of this book, the primary guideline will be the 2019 ACC/AHA Guideline on the Primary Prevention of Cardiovascular Disease. MEMBERS are volunteer scientists and healthcare professionals appointed by the leadership of the ACC and AHA.

AGATSTON SCORE - The Agatston score is a standardized scoring system for the Coronary Calcium Score.

AHA - American Heart Association

ACP (American College of Physicians) - The ACP is a national organization of internists, who specialize in the diagnosis, treatment, and care of adults.

Angiography, angiogram - angiography is the process. An angiogram is an image which is the same as cardiography or coronary angiogram.

Angioplasty - Angioplasty is the reconstruction of an artery. The term angiogram usually refers to using a coronary catheterization to clear a narrowed artery. This is also called PCI. See PCI.

Apolipoprotein - An apolipoprotein is the protein portion of a lipoprotein. Usually, lipoproteins consist of lipids and proteins bound together. Apolipoproteins are the protein portions without the lipid. See lipoprotein, LDL, and HDL.

Arteriography, arteriogram - Arteriography is the process of imaging an artery to understand the anatomy. This is most often done for concerns relating to CV disease. The purpose is to assess the distribution of plaque. Arteriogram is the image. It is the same as angiography, angiogram. See cardiography, cardiogram, or coronary angiogram.

Atherosclerosis - Atherosclerosis is the conditions of having plaque in the artery walls. It is also sometimes called arteriosclerosis.

Autophagy - This is a cellular biology term. It refers to the cell digesting and recycling deteriorated cellular materials for building blocks and energy. This first involves digesting these cellular parts into proteins, carbohydrates, and fats. The deteriorated (or senescent) materials include broken-down cell parts, such as mitochondria. (See Senescent and Mitochondria)

Biomarkers - Biomarkers are measurable substances in an organism whose presence is indicative of some phenomena such as disease, infection, or environmental exposure.

BMI (Body Mass Index) - BMI is an estimate of body fat based on height and weight. Many criticize BMI since it does not account for muscle. The risk factor is body fat, not muscle. The BMI typically underestimates fat mass in women and overestimates it in men. Arnold Schwarzenegger had a BMI of 30. His height was 6'2," and he weighed 235 pounds when he won the Mr. Olympia award. His body fat was only 8%. The "Schwarzenegger adjustment" of the BMI incorporates waist size. Some have proposed RFM (Relative Fat Mass) as a better estimate. It is not very well known. See RFM.

Cardiovascular (CV or CV) - Cardiovascular is a conflated term. The roots of the word imply heart and vascular disease. The real driver is arterial health. Arterial disease causes the vast majority of heart attacks, stroke, kidney, and eye disease. In other words, arterial health drives chronic diseases. Chronic diseases and aging are essentially arterial health problems. Arterial disease of the heart causes most deaths. Arterial disease impacting the brain causes most strokes (and maybe most dementia). CV disease is the biggest killer and disabler in the world. The majority of arterial disease is caused by insulin resistance (prediabetes or metabolic syndrome).

CAD (Coronary Atherosclerotic Disease) - CAD is the condition of having plaque in the arteries of the heart

Carotid Artery Sonography - See Carotid Ultrasound

Carotid B mode Ultrasound - Carotid B mode ultrasound refers to 'Brightness mode' in ultrasound. Brightness or B-mode is a black and white image which shows the tissue as reflected in B-mode. CIMT is conducted mostly in B-mode ultrasound. It uses a combination of ultrasound and information technology software to analyze the carotid artery wall.

Carotid Duplex Ultrasound - A Carotid Duplex includes both B-mode and Doppler studies.

Carotid Ultrasound - The use of ultrasound technology to examine the carotid artery or other tissues and organs in the body. This term alone does not differentiate between very different techniques: B-mode or brightness mode (which can look at artery wall structure) and Doppler (which features color movement of blood to evaluate at the velocity and directional flow of the blood). Duplex includes both B mode and Doppler.

Catabolic Metabolism - Catabolic metabolism breaks down or oxidizes materials. Autophagy is part of catabolic metabolism. Anabolic metabolism builds them up. (See Anabolic metabolism)

Cath angiogram - see coronary angiogram.

Catheter - A catheter is a thin, hollow tube. For purposes of this book, catheters are used for injecting Xray contrast dye into the arteries that supply the heart.

CHL/Quest- CHL(Cleveland Heart Labs) originally left Cleveland Clinic Labs to stand alone as a national lab focusing on specialized CV testing. CHL was purchased three years ago by Quest, a national general medical reference lab.

Cholesterol - Cholesterol is a waxy substance found in the blood. It is a crucial component of cell walls, hormones, vitamin D, brain cells, and bile (materials that help digest food). Cholesterol is a lipid. (See lipid)

Choosing Wisely - An educational campaign that involves contributing health information to Wikipedia. It is part of the Consumer Reports WikiProject and organized by the ABIM (American Board of Internal Medicine) Foundation. Choosing Wisely seeks to provide consumers and providers of healthcare services with information about health diagnostic procedures, which physicians frequently recommend despite a lack of evidence-based research demonstrating the usefulness of those procedures.

CIMT (Carotid Intima-Media Thickness) - A CIMT is a measurement of the thickness of the intima and media layers (the inner two layers) of the artery. A CIMT measurement is a direct measure of the inflammation in the arterial wall and can include the measurement of plaque (the result of long-term inflammation) in the arteries when present. The measurements are completed using ultrasound imaging technology and software analytics. It is a non-invasive, inexpensive, radiation-free and relatively simple test which generally takes less than 15 minutes of patient time and which requires no disrobing. It's also the only test that provides critical plaque characterization information which can tell patients and providers about the nature of the plaque (e.g. whether plaque is soft and vulnerable to rupture or dangerous, heterogenous which is slightly more stable, or calcified and completely healed). The CIMT suffers from a lack of standardization so individuals seeking a CIMT exam should be careful to select vendors with documented (peer-reviewed) data regarding reproducibility and protocol quality controls. We discuss how to overcome this disadvantage. It can be used to monitor efficacy of treatment and had been shown to be reproducible to 0.002mm.

Cohort - A cohort is any group that shares an experience. The term is used to describe studies like Framingham that follow populations through an experience or period of time.

CAD - CAD is an acronym for Coronary Artery Disease.

Coronary Angiogram - A Coronary Angiogram is a procedure that uses dye injected into the heart's arteries for Xray imaging. The injection is usually done using a catheter inserted into the femoral artery at the groin and threaded up through the aorta to the heart. Other names include coronary artery angiogram, cath angiogram, heart catheterization, cardiac cath.

Coronary Artery Calcium Score (or calcium score) – A Coronary Calcium Score is a measurement of calcium in the arteries of the heart using CT imaging. The presence of any calcium indicates there is plaque in these arteries. This test is easily accessible, inexpensive, and well standardized. It is a great screen. But it is not great for tracking progress (monitoring).

CRP (C-Reactive Protein) - CRP is a protein made by the liver in reaction to many types of inflammation. Because elevated CRP is consistently associated with CV disease, including heart attack and stroke, it is an important biomarker - or predictor - of heart attacks. The inflammation measured can start from any type of cell damage, ranging from burns to cuts to flu shots so it is not specific to CV disease. The biggest problem with CRP is that elevated levels can be due to these other types of injuries and not just heart disease. For example, two days after a flu shot, 66% of patients have CRP elevation.

CTA (Computerized Tomography Angiogram) – CTA is a measurement and imaging of plaque and anatomy of the coronary arteries using intravenous Xray dye and CT imaging. Recent studies indicate this could bring much clarity to the usual stress testing. There has been a rapid "learning curve," resulting in the need to encourage the use of the CTA and the use of the latest equipment to avoid radiation.

Cytokines – Any of several substances, such as interleukin, interferon, and growth factors which are secreted by certain cells of the immune system and have an effect on other cells.

CV (also CV, cardiovascular) - CV means relating to the heart and blood vessels. CV is a confusing term. It is rooted in a conflated concept (cardiac vs. vascular) See cardiovascular.

CVD - CVD is an acronym for Coronary Vascular Disease. It also sometimes means the more general term Cardiovascular Disease.

Doppler Ultrasound - A Doppler ultrasound of an artery estimates flow based on changes in frequency (pitch). Doppler studies measure velocity and direction of flow, not plaque. Most heart attacks (86%) occur in individuals with insufficient plaque to cause blood flow abnormalities or hemodynamic changes.

Embolism - An embolism is the process of a blockage-causing piece of material, inside a blood vessel. The embolus may be a blood clot (thrombus), a fat globule (fat embolism), a bubble of air or other gas (gas embolism), or foreign material. (See embolus and thrombus)

Embolus - An embolus is a blood clot, air bubble, piece of fatty deposit, or other object which has been carried in the bloodstream to lodge in a vessel and cause an infarction, or tissue death. (See thrombus)

Framingham Risk Calculator - a predictive equation developed from the Framingham Heart Study. The ACC/AHA Preventive standards committee recommends that doctors initiate a CV risk evaluation using a Framingham risk estimator. The Framingham equation incorporates demographics such as age, gender, and race. Other CV risk factors are included as well, such as smoking. Different Framingham risk calculators vary in the list of risk factors they include.

Glycocalyx – Literally means "sugar coat" (glykys = sweet, kalyx = husk). A network of polysaccharides that project from cellular surfaces of bacteria, which classifies it as a universal surface component of a bacterial cell, found just outside the bacterial cell wall.

HDL (High-Density Lipoprotein) - Some people still call HDL the "good" cholesterol because higher levels are markers for decreased CV risk. HDL carries cholesterol from other parts of the body back to the liver for removal in a process known as 'Reverse Cholesterol Transport'. HDL includes cholesterol and a different carrier protein from LDL.

Haptoglobin 2 - This is a genetic variation of haptoglobin. Usually, haptoglobin clears arteries of deteriorated, oxidized hemoglobin. Haptoglobin 2 is deficient in this vital role. That appears to have created an advantageous resistance to malaria for carriers of haptoglobin 2. The trade-off is accelerated oxidation (inflammation) of tissues like artery walls. The precursor molecule (zonulin) causes other inflammatory diseases, such as leaky gut and Hashimoto's thyroiditis.

Heart catheterization - see coronary catheterization.

Hemoglobin A1c (also called A1c or glycated hemoglobin) - your hemoglobin with glucose attached. The A1c test evaluates the average amount of glucose in the blood over the last 2 to 3 months by measuring the percentage of glycated hemoglobin in the blood.

Homeostasis – In biology and physiology, homeostasis is the steady state maintained in the internal, physical, and chemical conditions maintained by living systems. It is the condition of optimal function for the organism which includes many variables such as body temperature, fluid balance being kept within certain pre-set limits.

hsCRP - high sensitivity CRP. An hsCRP is simply a CRP test showing much lower levels of CRP than the original CRP measurement. CRP ranges from 10 to 1,000 mg/L, whereas hsCRP values range from .5 to 10 mg/L. For this book, we use the terms interchangeably.

IF (Intermittent Fasting) - Abstaining from food for various periods. Most people are referring to the practice of skipping breakfast when they use the term Intermittent Fasting. It can also mean TRE. OMAD is also a form of IF. (See OMAD and TRE)

IMT (intima-media Thickness) - IMT measurements can be taken on virtually any vascular bed. CIMT refers to those IMT measurements in the Carotid arteries. IMT measurements have been taken in the femoral and other arteries (see CIMT). Although IMT is generally measured off ultrasound images, it can also be measured from Intravascular Ultrasound, MRI, and other imaging modalities.

Infarction - Loss of blood supply due to an organ or region of tissue, usually by an embolus or thrombus

Inflammation - Inflammation is a vital part of the immune system's response to injury and infection. It involves signaling and defense coordinated by multiple immune cell lines, enzymes, and biomarkers. (See Inflammation panel, CRP, LP-PLA2, and MPO)

Inflammation Panel - An inflammation panel is a panel of tests used to measure inflammation. In this book, we are referring to our preferred panel, developed by CHL, now part of Quest national labs. It includes hsCRP, Lp-PLA2, MPO, and MACR.

Interleukin 6 (IL6) - IL6 is a protein (and gene) associated with inflammation. Rheumatoid arthritis and Kaposi's sarcoma are associated with increased IL6. IL6 is also a biomarker for CV inflammation.

Invasive angiography, angiogram - see angiogram. The differentiating term here is "invasive." It means this angiogram was done as part of a cardiac cath procedure, not as a simple CT angiogram.

IR (Insulin Resistance) - The decreased response of the muscle and liver cell membrane to insulin receptors. IR leads to an inability to get sugar out of the blood and into the cell, where it does less damage. IR is the most common cause of CV inflammation and plaque. Also called Prediabetes or Metabolic Syndrome. (There are some slight technical differences, but they are not significant for this book.) IR can lead to diabetes, CV inflammation, plaque, heart attack, stroke, dementia, blindness, erectile dysfunction, and other chronic diseases associated with aging.

IVUS - Intravascular Ultrasound. Use of Ultrasound to create images of arterial plaque from inside the artery during an invasive cardiac cath procedure. This procedure is still investigational. It is beyond the scope of this book.

Insulin Response - this is a term for a test of insulin values added to each glucose measurement in an OGTT. An insulin response study tells the amount of insulin required to achieve a blood sugar level.

Insulin Survey - an OGTT with an Insulin Response. There are different values and forms of these tests. The two most common, for purposes of this book, are the Insulin Survey done through Quest labs for Dr. Brewer's clinic and the Kraft Insulin Survey. Both tests include an OGTT, which is at least 8 hours fasting followed by a glucose challenge and serial measurements of blood glucose and insulin levels. The Quest test uses 75 grams of glucose and measures blood glucose and insulin at 1 and 2 hours. The Kraft insulin survey typically uses 100 grams of glucose followed by blood glucose and insulin tests at 30 minutes and 1, 2, 3, and 4 hours.

Ischemia or ischeamia - Ischemia is restriction of blood supply to tissues, causing a shortage of oxygen. Cell metabolism requires oxygen. Ischemia is generally caused by problems with blood vessels, with resultant damage to or dysfunction of tissue. ISCHEMIA is also the name of a recent randomized clinical trial that demonstrated bypass grafts do not prevent heart attack.

JACC - Journal of the American College of Cardiology

kDa(kiloDalton) - a measure of molecular weight

Kraft Insulin Survey - The Kraft Insulin Survey is one of the best methods measuring insulin resistance. It is similar to an OGTT, but it includes insulin measurements at all the blood glucose checks. The Kraft survey also uses 100 grams of glucose instead of 75. And it typically goes three or four hours instead of two. (See OGTT)

LDL (Low-Density Lipoprotein) - LDL is sometimes called "bad" cholesterol because oxidized forms of LDL are the primary component of arterial plaque. Cholesterol is a type of fat or lipid. LDL doesn't mix well with blood serum, which is 90% water, so the body makes proteins to bind lipids for transport in the serum. HDL cholesterol includes cholesterol and a different protein.

Lipid - The term lipid is a class of compounds including fats, waxes, and oils. Lipids are organic, meaning carbon-based. They dissolve in other carbon-based compounds, but not water. They are major components of the body. The body has made proteins to transport lipids such as cholesterol within the body. (See lipoproteins, cholesterol, LDL)

Lipoproteins - proteins made by the body to transport lipids

Lp-PLA2 (LipoProtein - associated PhosphoLipase A2) is an enzyme that plays a role in CV inflammation. It is released by a family of immune cells (mast cells, macrophages, T cells, and foam cells) to break down plaque.

For medical scientists - It hydrolyzes oxidized phospholipids in LDL. The PLA2G7 gene codes it. It is a 45 kDa protein made of 441 amino acids. In the blood, it travels mainly with LDL. Less than 20% is associated with HDL.

A meta-analysis involving 29,036 participants in 32 prospective studies found that Lp-PLA2 levels correlate with increased risk of coronary heart disease and stroke. (Thompson 2010)

Lumen - A lumen is an opening, the inside space of a tubular structure. The lumen is the inside of the arterial tube. CV plaque is commonly assumed to be inside the lumen of the artery, but over 90% of the plaque grows away from the lumen and into the arterial wall.

Oxidized LDL gets trapped between the inside layer (intima) and the middle layer (media). This specific location is essential because it leads to the inability to predict heart attack and stroke. The mechanism of most heart attacks and strokes involves liquid plaque escaping from the artery wall and causing a clot inside the lumen of the artery.

MACR (Microalbumin Creatinine Ratio) - a measurement of microscopic amounts of the protein albumin in the urine. Albumin is a major protein usually present in the blood, but virtually no albumin is present in the urine when the kidneys are functioning correctly. MACR is used to screen for kidney disease in people with chronic diseases such as hypertension or diabetes. Microalbuminuria is an independent and robust indicator of increased CV risk among individuals with and without diabetes. (Stehouwer 2006)

MESA Score - The Multi-Ethnic Study of Atherosclerosis (MESA) score is a CV risk calculator. You can find it at (https://www.mesa-nhlbi.org/calcium/input.aspx). It incorporates CAC score in addition to the traditional risk factors of demographics, cholesterol, systolic blood pressure, diabetes, smoking, family history of CHD, and the use of hypertension or cholesterol medications. The MESA calculator is a result of the study of the same name. (Budoff 2009)

Meta-analysis - A meta-analysis is a study that looks at many other studies conducted on a particular subject. Meta-analysis papers (also called literature reviews or lit reviews) are systematic reviews regarding the available or published science in a field of study.

Metabolic Syndrome - see Insulin Resistance and Prediabetes.

Mitochondria - Mitochondria are the powerhouses or furnaces of the cell. Mitochondria burn energy sources.

MPO (Myeloperoxidase) - MPO is an enzyme released by a family of immune cells to carry out antimicrobial activity. It is part of the CHL/Quest CV Inflammation panel, along with CRP, LP-PLA2, and MACR. Myelo means bone marrow, and peroxidase is a type of enzyme. MPO has a green heme pigment component leading to the greenish color of mucus. MPO blood levels indicate the risk of coronary artery disease. (Zhang 2001)

For doctors - MPO is a peroxidase encoded by the MPO gene on chromosome 17. It produces acids to carry out an antimicrobial activity. It is a 150 kDa protein consisting of two 15 kDa light chains and two glycosylated heavy chains bound to a prosthetic heme group.

MPI (Myocardial Perfusion Imaging) - Myocardial perfusion imaging (MPI) is a non-invasive imaging test that shows how well blood flows through (perfuses) your heart muscle. It can show areas of the heart muscle that are not getting enough blood flow. This test is often called a nuclear stress test.

Myocardium - Myocardium is the muscle of the heart. The prefix myo means muscle.

NCEP (The National Cholesterol Education Program) - The NCEP is a program managed by the National Heart, Lung, and Blood Institute, a division of the National Institutes of Health. Its goal is "to reduce increased cardiovascular disease rates due to hypercholesterolemia (elevated cholesterol levels) in the United States of America." The program has been running since 1985.

Nomogram - A nomogram is a graphical calculation tool. The only one used in this book is the standard IMT measurement for men and women by age.

OGTT (Oral Glucose Tolerance Test) - A test for Insulin Resistance. The OGTT is a measurement of Insulin Resistance. There are multiple types. All involve fasting for eight hours, followed by a glucose challenge and then serial measurements of blood glucose. The OGTT measures the body's ability to metabolize carbohydrates. The most common problem is the resistance of the insulin receptors in the muscle and liver cell membranes.

IR leads to prediabetes, diabetes, CV inflammation, plaque, heart attack, stroke, dementia, blindness, erectile dysfunction, and other chronic diseases associated with aging. The Kraft Insulin Survey is a more detailed test, adding insulin levels to all blood sugar tests. Most Kraft Insulin Surveys also use 100 grams of glucose instead of 75. (See also Kraft Insulin Survey)

OMAD - One Meal per Day. A popular method for weight loss. It also closes the feeding or eating window. OMAD tends to decrease caloric intake. It also stimulates the body to switch back and forth between catabolic and anabolic metabolism. Satchin Panda, Valter Longo, and others have recently demonstrated that this switching improves health. (See Catabolic, Anabolic, Autophagy, IF and TRE).

PCI (Percutaneous Coronary Intervention) - A PCI is the process of using a catheter to clear a narrowed artery of the heart. (See Stent or Angioplasty)

Perfusion - Perfusion is the passage of blood, a blood substitute, or other fluid through the blood vessels or other natural channels in an organ or tissue.

PET (Positron Emission Tomography) - A PET scan is a process of using a radioactive tracer to generate images tending to be more detailed than other nuclear imaging tests. See stress tests.

Plaque - A plaque is a distinct region of damage to the intimal lining of the artery resulting from deposits of necrotic (dead) material, active macrophages, and other enzymes and cytokines.

Plaques are generally found within the walls of arteries, not in the lumen, but in their final stages, the pimple-like lesion grows into the lumen or inside of the artery. The term plaque is often used in related fields of study: dentistry and study of Alzheimer's dementia.

In dentistry, these plaques are made mostly of bacterial residues. In Alzheimer's and dementia, the plaques are made of a protein called beta-amyloid.

Prediabetes - See Insulin Resistance

Reactive Hyperemia – A transient increase in organ blood flow that occurs following a brief period of ischemia or arterial occlusion (blockage).

RFM (Relative Fat Mass) - RFM is another method of estimating fat mass suggested as a better option than the BMI. It uses only waist circumference and height. It was developed using NHANES data. It avoids the typical BMI errors of underestimating fat mass in women and overestimating it in men.

Sarcopenia - Loss of muscle mass. The root sarco means muscle, and the root penia means loss. Sarcopenia is strongly related to age beyond 65 years, inflammation, prediabetes, and death.

Senescence - The condition or process of deterioration with age.

Sensitivity - Sensitivity is a test characteristic. Sensitivity is the ability to identify those with the disease correctly. It is also called the true positive rate. That is the percentage of true positive test results divided by all tested. (See Specificity)

Serum - Serum is the liquid part of the blood.

Specificity - Specificity is a test characteristic. Specificity is the ability to identify those without the disease correctly. It is also called the true negative rate. That is the percentage of true negative test results divided by all tested.

SPECT (Single Photon Emission Computerized Tomography) - SPECT is a process of using a radioactive tracer to generate images tending to be more detailed than other nuclear imaging tests. See stress tests.

Stress Test - A stress test is a procedure used to measure how the heart works during physical activity. These typically involve assessment of heart function while exercising on a treadmill, exercise bike, or during drug-induced heart stress.

Stress tests are by far the most common method of looking for cardiovascular risk. They have many problems, such as high false positive and false negative tests when used to predict heart attack and stroke. Even conservative standards bodies like the American College of Cardiology, the Internal Medicine Foundation, and the American College of Family Practitioners agree that doctors and patients are using too many stress tests.

Researchers have developed multiple ways of assessing heart function during the test to improve the stress test. Examples include EKG, physical symptoms such as breathlessness and fatigue, echo/ultrasound, and multiple forms involving radiation such as MRI, SPECT, and PET scans.

Thrombus - A thrombus is a blood clot formed in situ within the vascular system of the body and impeding blood flow.

TRF (Time-Restricted Feeding) or TRE (Time-Restricted Eating) - TRF or TRE are acronyms referring to narrowing the time of day for caloric input. This tends to decrease caloric intake. It also stimulates the body to switch back and forth between catabolic and anabolic metabolism. Satchin Panda, Valter Longo, and others have recently demonstrated that this switching improves health. (Longo 2016).

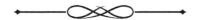

BIBLIOGRAPHY

AAFP. (2012). 2012 AAFP recommendations for preventive services guideline. 08-2005.

ADA. (2018). Classification and Diagnosis of Diabetes: Standards of Medical Care in Diabetes. *Diabetes Care*, 41(Supplement 1):S13-S27.

Agatston, A. (2016). *Youtube*, Vidio Source: https://www.youtube.com/watch?v=Q31ltU_U-jE.

Al-Lamee, R. T. (2018). Percutaneous coronary intervention in stable angina (ORBITA): a double-blind, randomized controlled trial. *The Lancet*, 391:10115-31-40.

Allan, P. M. (1997, February). Relationship Between Carotid Intima-Media Thickness and Symptomatic and Asymptomatic Peripheral Arterial Disease. *Stroke*, 28(2), 348-. doi:10.1161/01.STR.28.2.348

Arbab-Zadeh, A. (2012). Stress testing and non-invasive coronary angiography in patients with sustpected coronary artery disease: time for a new paradigm. *Heart International*, 7(1), e2, DOI:10.4081/hi.2012.e2.

Arnett, D. B. (2019). ACC/AHA Guideline on the Primary Prevention of Cardiovascular Disease: A Report of the American College of Cardiology / American Heart Association Task Force on Clinical Practice Guidelines. *Circulation*, 140(11).

Babey SH, W. J. (2016). Prediabetes in California: Nearly Half of California Adults on Path to Diabetes. UCLA Fielding School of Publich Health Policy Brief: *https://healthpolicy.ucla.edu/publications/search/pages/detail.aspx?PubID=1472.*

Bakalar, N. (March 16, 2015). Too Much Cardiac Testing. *New York Times.*

Bale B, D. A. (2014). *Beat the Heart Attack Gene.* Nashville, TN: Wiley General Trade, an imprint of Turner Publishing Company .

Bartels, S. F. (2012). Carotid intima-media thickness (cIMT) and plaque from risk assessment and clinical use to genetic discoveries. *Perspective in Medicine,* 1, 139-145.

Becaro, G. N. (2001). Carotid and femoral ultrasound morphology screening and cardiovascular events in low risk subjects: a 10-year follow-up study (the CAFES-CAVE study). *Atheroslcerosis,* 156, 379-387. doi:10.1016/S0021-9150(00)00665-1

Berk, B. W. (1990). Elevaton of C-Reactive Protein In "Active" Coronary Artery Disease. *Am J Cardiol,* 65:168-172.

Blaha, M. M. (2017). Coronary Artery Calcium Scoring. Is it Time for a Change in Methodology? *JACC,* Imaging.10(8).

Boden, W.O. (2007). The Evolving Pattern of Symptomatic Coronary Artery Disease in the United States and Canada: Baseline Characteristics of the Clinical Outcomes Utilizing Revascularization and Aggressive Drug Evaluation (COURAGE) Trial. *The American Journal of Cardiology,* 208-212.

Bonithon-Kopp, C. T. (1996, February). Relation of Intima-Media Thickness to Atherosclerotic Plaques in Carotid Arteries: The Vascular Aging (EVA) Study. *Arteriosclerosis, Thrombosis, and Vascular Biology,* 16(2), 310-316. doi:10.1161/01.ATV.16.2.310

Bots, M. H. (1997). Common carotid intima-media thickness and risk of stroke and myocardial infarction: the Rotterdam Study. *Circulation,* 96(5), 1432-1437.

Budoff, M. (2006). Assessment of Coronary Artery Disease by Cardiac Computed Tomography. *Circulation,* 114:1761-1791.

Budoff, M. (2009). Coronary Calcium predicts events better with absolute calcium scores than age-gender-race percentiles - the Multi-Ethnic Study of Atherosclerosis (MESA). *JACC,* Jan 27;53(4) 345-352.

Budoff, M. M. (2017). Prognostic Value of Coronary Artery Calcium in the PROMISE Study (Prospective Multicenter Imaging Study for Evaluation of

Chest Pain). *Circulation*, 136:1993-2005.

Campbell, T., & TM., C. (2004). The China Study: Startling Implications For Diet, Weight Loss And Long-Term Health. In T. Campbell, & C. TM., *The China Study: Startling Implications For Diet, Weight Loss And Long-Term Health*. Dallas, TX.: BenBella Books, Inc.

Carpeggiani, C. (2017). Variability of radiation doses of cardiac diagnostic imaging tests: the RADIO-EVINCI study (RADIation dOse suproject of the EVINCI study). *BMC Cardiovascular Disorder*, 17(63).

Carovac, A. S. (2011, June 1st). Application of Ultrasound in Medicine. *AIM*, 19(3), 168-171.

Carroll, A. (2018). Heart Stents Are Useless for Most Stable Patients. They're Still Widely Used. Why Are So Many People Agreeing To An Expensive Procedure - and Putting Themselves At Risk for a Placebo Effect? *New York Times*, Feb 12,.

Carroll, A. (April 15, 2016). A Study on Fats That Doesn't Fit the Story Line. *The New York Times*.

Casey DE, T. R. (2019). AHA/ACC Clinical Performance and Quality Measures for Adults With High Blood Pressure. *Circulation*, 12:e000057.

CDC. (July 18, 2017). New CDC Report: More Than 100 Million Americans Have Diabetes Or Prediabetes. *Press Release*.

Chambless, L. H. (1997). Association of Coronary Heart Disease Incidence with Carotid Arterial Wall Thickness and Major Risk Factors: The Atherosclerosis Risk in Communities (ARIC) Study, 1987 - 1993. *American Journal of Epidemiology*, 146(6), 483-494.

Chambless, L. F. (2000). Carotid Wall Thickness is Predictive of Incident Clinical Stroke. (J. H. Health, Ed.) *American Journal of Epidemiology*, 151(5), 478-487.

Cheng, H. G. (2016). Effect of comprehensive cardiovascular disease risk management on longitudinal changes in carotid artery intima-media thickness in a community-based prevention clinic. *Arch Med Sci*, 12(4)728-735.

Chou, R. (2015). High-Value Care Task Force of the American College of Physicians. Cardiac Screening With Electrocardiography, Stress

Echocardiography, or Myocardial Perfusion Imaging: Advice for High-Value Care From the American College of Physicians. *Ann Intern Med*, 162: 438-447.

Cook, N. R. (2014). Futher insight into the cardiovascular risk calculator: the roles of statins, revascularizations, and underascertainment in the Women's Health Study. *JAMA*, 174(12)1964-1971. DOI:10.1001/jamainternmed.2014.5336.

Costanzo, P. P.-F. (2010). Does Carotid Intima-Media Thickness Regression Predict Reduction of Cardiovascular Events? A Meta-Analysis of 41 Randomized Trials. *JACC*, 56(24): 2006-20.

Crouse, J. R. (2007). Effect of Rosuvastatin on Progression of Carotid Intima-Media Thickness in Low-Risk Individuals With Subclinical Atherosclerosis. *JAMA*, 297(12), 1344-1353.

Cummins, I. G. (2018). Eat Rich, Live Long. Las Vegas, NV.: *Victory Belt Publishing Inc.*

Currie, G. D. (2014). Proteinuria and its relation to cardiovascular disease. *Int J Nephrol Renovasc Dis*, 7:13-24.

Curzen, N. S. (2005). Consent in cardiology: there may be trouble ahead? *Heart*, Jul;91(7)977-80.

DeCabo, R. M. (2019). Effects of Intermittent Fasting on Health, Aging, and Disease. *NEJM*, 381:2541-2551.

Diehm, C. S. (2004). High prevalence of peripheral arterial disease and comorbidity in 6880 primary care patients: a cross-sectional study. *Atherosclerosis*, 172:95-105.

DiFrancesco, A. D. (2018). A time to fast. *Science*, 362:770-775.

Disruption, C. P. (1995). E Falk, PK Shah, V Fuster. . ;. *Circulation*, 92:657.

Douglas, P. H. (2014). PROspective Multicenter Imaging Study for Evaluation of chest pain: Rationale and design of the PROMISE trial. *American Heart Journal*, 796-803.e1.

Einstein, A. P. (2015). INCAPS Investigators Group. Current worldwide nuclear cardiology practices and radiation exposure: results from the 65 country IAEA Nuclear Cardiology Protocols Cross-Sectional Study (INCAPS). *Eur Heart J.*, 36(26): 1689-1696.

Elias-Smale, S. K. (2011). Common carotid intima-media thickness in cardiovascular risk stratification of older people: the Rotterdam Study. *European Journal of Preventative Cardiology*, 19(4), 698-705.

E Falk, P. S. (1995). Coronary plaque disruption. *Circulation*, 225-324.

Falk, E. S. (1995). Coronary Plaque Disruption. *Circulation*, 92:657-671.

Fasano, A. S.-D. (2005). Mechanisms of Disease: the role of intestinal barrier function in the pathogenesis of gastrointestinal diseases. *Nature Clinical Practice, Gastroenterology & Hepatology 2*, 416-422.

Feigelson HS, C. M. (1994). Screening for peripheral arterial disease: the sensitivity, specificity, and predictive value of non-invasive tests in a defined population. *Am J Epidemiol*, 140:526-34.

Garber A.M., S. N. (1999). Cost-effectiveness of alternative test strategies for the diagnosis of coronary artery disease." ;. *Annals of Internal Medicine.*, 130(9):719.

Gawande, A. (2009). The Cost Conundrum. *The New Yorker*.

Gibbons, R. e. (1997). Guidelines for Exercise Testing. A Report of the American College of Cardiology / American Heart Association Task Force on Practice Guidelines (Committee on Exercise Testing). *JACC*, Vol. 30, No. 1 July 1997:260-315.

Gilbert, E. (2010). Ionizing Radiation and Cancer Risks: What Have We Learned From Epidemiology? *Int J Radiat Biol*, 85(6): 467-482.

Gina Kolata. (2013). Risk Calculator for Cholesterol Appears Flawed. *New York Times*, https://www.nytimes.com/2013/11/18/health/risk-calculator-for-cholesterol-appears-flawed.html.

Gluckman, T. L. (2019). 8 Million Nuclear Stress Tests are Performed in the US. Is This Necessary? *Oliver Wyman*, https://health.oliverwyman.com/2019/04/-is-this-necessary----some-docs-order-too-many-expensive--danger.html.

Gogg, D. e. (2014). Guideline on the Assessment of Cardiovascular Risk. *JACC*, 63(25):2935-59.

Goldberg, E. M. (2019). Coronary Artery Calcium Score in Decision Making: the MESA score. *Lipids*, https://www.lipid.org/node/1899.

Goldstein JL, Brown MS. A century of cholesterol and coronaries: from plaques to genes to statins. *Cell*. 2015;161(1):161–172. doi:10.1016/j.cell.2015.01.036

Greenland, P. A. (2000). Prevention Conference V: Beyond Secondary Prevention: Identifying the High-Risk Patient for Primary Prevention. Noninvasive Tests of Atherosclerotic Burden. Writing Group III. *Circulation*, 101, e16-e22.

Greenland, P. A. J. (2010). 2010 ACCF/AHA guideline for assessment of cardiovascular risk in asymptomatic adults: executive summary. *J Am Coll Cardiol*, 56:.2182-2199.

Grundy, S. S. (2018). AHA/ACC/AACVPR/AAPA/ABC/ACPM/ADA/AGS/ APhA/ASPC/NLA Guideline on the management of blood cholesterol: a report of the American College of Cardiology/American Heart Associaton Tast Force on Practice Guidelines. *JACC*.

Hanson, H. V. (2018). Prevalence of Carotid Plaque in a 63- to 65- Year Old Norwegian Cohort From the General Population: The ACE 1950 Study. *Journal of the American Heart Association (AHA)*, 1-9.

Harvard University. (2006). Sudden Death Isn't Always So Sudden. *Harvard Heart Letter*.

Hendel RC, B. D. (2009). 2009 appropriate use criteria for cardiac radionuclide imaging: a report of the American College of Cardiology Foundation Appropriate Use Criteria Task Force, the American Society of Nuclear Cardiology, the American College of Radiology, the American Hear. *J Am Coll Cardiol*, 53:2201–29.

Henry, R., Ferreira, I., & al., e. (2004). Type 2 diabetes is associated with impaired endothelium-dependent, flow-mediated dilation, but impaired glucose metabolism is not. The Hoorn Study. *Atherosclerosis*, 49-56.

Herman, A. (2019). ISCHEMIA: Invasive Treatment Not Better Than Meds in Patients with Stable Ischemic Heart Disease. *NEJM*, NEJM Journal Watch Nov 18.

Hiatt. (2001). Medical Treatment of Peripheral Arterial Disease and Claudication. *NEJM*. 344:1608-1621.

Hoffmann, U. F. (2017). Prognostic Value of Noninvasive Cardiovascular Testing in Patients With Stable Chest Pain: Insights From the PROMISE Trial (Prospective Multicenter Imaging Study for Evaluation of Chest Pain). *Circulation*, 135:2320-2332 www.ahajournals.org/doi/10.1161/CIRCULATIONAHA.116.024360.

Honda, O. S. (2004). Echolucent Carotid Plaques Predict Future Coronary Events in Patients With Coronary Artery Disease. *JACC*, 43(7):1177-84.

Huang L., C. K. (2019). SR-B1 Drives Endothelial Cell LDL Transcytosis via DOCK4 to Promote Atherosclerosis. *Nature*, 569, 565-569 DOE:10.1038/s41586-019-1140-4.

Khan, T. F. (2008). Critical Review of the Ankle Brachial Index. *Curr Cardiol Rev*, 4(2)101-106.

Iglesias del Sol, A. (2001). *CArdiovascular risk assessment using carotid ultrasonography: The Rotterdam Study*. Erasmus University Rotterdam. doi: 978-90-77017-09-8

Ioannidis, J. (2005). Why Most Published Research Findings Are False. *PLOS Med*, 2(8): e124.

Kawagishi, T., & Matsuyoshi, M. e. (1999). Impaired endothelium-dependent vascular responses of retinal and intrarenal arteries in patients with type 2 diabetes. *Atheroscler Throm Basc Biol*, 19:2509-2516.

Kolata, G. (2013). Risk Calculator for Cholesterol Appears Flawed. *New York Times*, https://www.nytimes.com/2013/11/18/health/risk-calculator-for-cholesterol-appears-flawed.html.

Kraft, J. (2008). *The Diabetes Epidemic and You*. Bloomington, IN.: Trafford Publishing.

Ladapo, J. B. (2014). Physician Decision Making and Trends in the Use of Cardiac Stress Testing in the United States: An Analysis of Repeated Cross-Sectional Data. *Intern Med*, 161(7):482-490.A.

Lavie, C. M. (2008). The Russert Impact: A Golden Opportunity to Promote Primary Coronary Prevention. *The Ochsner Journal*, 8:108-113.

Liuzzo G, B. L. (1994). The Prognostic Value of C-Reactive Protein and Serum Amyloid A Protein In Severe Unstable Angina. *N Engl J Med*, 342:836-843.

Loannidis, J. (2005). Why Most Published Research Findings Are False. *PLoS Med*, 2(8): e124.

Longo, V. M. (2014). Fasting: molecular mechanisms and clinical applications. *Cell Metab*, 19:181-192.

Longo, V. P. (2016). Fasting, Circadian Rhythms, and Time-Restricted Feeding in Healthy Lifespan. . *Cell Metabolism*, 23(6): 1048-1059.

Loop, F. (1987). F. Mason Sones, Jr., M.D. (1918 - 1985). *Ann Thorac Surg*, 43:237-238 https://www.annalsthoracicsurgery.org/article/S0003-4975(10)60411-0/pdf.

Ludwig, D. (2016). *Always Hungry*. New York, NY: Grand Central Publishing, Hachette Book Group.

Manda, Y. B., (2018). Cardiac Catheterization, Risks, and Complications. *StatPearls*, Bookshelf ID: NBK531461PMID: 30285356, https://www.ncbi.nlm.nih.gov/books/NBK531461/.

Meng, S. F. (2015). Monocytes and Macrophages in Atherosclerosis. In H. P. Wang, *Atherosclerosis. Risks, Mechanisms and Therapies*. (pp. 141-154). Philadelphia, PA: John Wiley & Sons, Inc.

Mercuri, M. P. (2016). Comparison of Radiation Doses and Best-Practice Use for Myocardial Perfusion Imaging in the US and Non-US Laboratories: Findings From the IAEA (International Atomic Energy Agency) Nuclear Cardiology Protocols Study. *JAMA*, 176(2):266-269.

Mercuri, M. P. (2016). Estimating the Reduction in the Radiation Burden From Nuclear Cardiology Through Use of Stress-Only Imaging in the United States and Worldwide. *JAMA Intern Med*, 176(2): 269-273.

Merriam-Webster. (2019). Definition of 'Cohort'. *Internet*, hpps://www.merriam-webster.com/dictionary/cohort.

Messenger, B. L. (2016). Coronary calcium scans and radiation exposure in the multi-ethnic study of atherosclerosis. *Int J Cardiovasc Imaging*, 32: 525.

Mettler, F. W. (2008). Effective Doses in Radiology and Diagnostic Nuclear Medicine: A Catalog 1. *Radiology*, 248(1):254-63.

Moussa, I. H. (2013). The NCDR CathPCI Registry: a US national perspective on care and outcomes for percuanious coronary intervention. *Heart*, Mar;99(5):297-303 DOI:10.1136/heartjnl-2012-303379.

Meyer, J. (1990). Werner Forssmann and Catheterization of the Heart, 1929. *Ann Thorac Surg*, 49:497-9.

Mohler, E. G.-H. (2012). ACCF/ACR/AIUM/ASE/ASN/ICAVL/SCAI/SCCT/SIR/SVM/SVS 2012 Appropriate Use Criteria for Peripheral Vascular Ultrasound and Physiological Testing Part I: Arterial Ultrasound and Physiological Testing. *JACC*, 60(3):242-76.

Moyer, V. (2012). U.S. Preventive Services Task Force. Screening for coronary heart disease with electrocardiography: U.S. Preventive Services Task Force recommendation statement. *Ann Intern Med*, 512-518.

Murabito, J. E. (2003). The Ankle-Brachial Index in the Elderly and Risk of Stroke, Coronary Disease, and Death. *JAMA*, 163(16):1939-1942.

Naghavi, M. F. (2006). The first SHAPE (Screening for Heart Attack Prevention and Education) guideline. *Crit Pathw Cardiol*, 5(4): 187-90.

Nemetz PN, R. V. (2008). Recent trends in the prevalence of cornoary disease: a population-based autopsy study of nonnatrual deaths. *Arch Intern Med*, 168:264-70.

Newby, D. W. (2015). CT coronary angiography in patients with suspected angina due to coronary heart disease (SCOT-HEART): an open-label, parallel-group, multicentre trial. *The Lancet*, Pages 2383-2391.

O'Hare, A. K. (2006). Mortality and cardiovascular risk across the ankle-arm index spectrum: results from the Cardiovascular Health Study. Circulation. *Circulation*, 113:388-93.

O'Leary, D. P. (1999). Carotid-artery intima and media thickness as a risk factor for myocardial infarction and stroke in older adults. *N Engl J Med*, 340(1), 14-22

Oshima K, H. S. (2017). More than a biomarker: the systemic consequences of heparan sulfate fragments released during endothelial surface layer degradation. *Pulm Circ*, 8(1).

Perez, H. G. (2016). Adding carotid total plaque area to the Framingham risk score improves cardiovascular risk classification. *Arch Med Sci*, 12(3):513-520.

Pignoli, P. (1984). Ultrasound B-mode imaging for arterial wall thickness measurement. *Atherosclerosis Reviews*, 12, 177-184.

Pignoli, P. T. (1986). Intimal plus medial thickness of the arterial wall: a direct measurement with ultrasound imaging. *Circulation*, 6(74), 1399-1406. doi:10.1161/01.cir.74.6.1399

Qamruddin, S. (2016). False-Positive Stress Echocardiograms: A continuing Challenge. *The Oshsner JI.*, 16(3):277-279.

Riches, N. A. (2010). Standardized ultrasound protocol, trained sonographers, and digital system for carotid atherosclerosis screening. *J.Cardiovac Med*, 11(9):683-688.

Ridker PM, C. M. (1997). Inflammation, Asparin, and The Risk of Cardiovascular Disease in Apparently Healthy Men. *N Engl J Med*, 336:973-979.

Ridker PM. (2015). A Test in Context: High-Sensitivity C-Reactive Protein. *JACC*, 67:6.

Roberts, R. S. (2012). 9p21 and the genetic revolution for coronary artery disease. *Clinical Chemistry*, 104-12.

Rospleszcz, S. T. (2019). Temporal trends in cardiovascular risk factors and performance of the Framingham Risk Score and the Pooled Cohort Equations. *J Epidemiol Community Health*, 73:19-25.

Rozanski, A. (2011). Impact of Coronary Artery Calcium Scanning on Coronary Risk Factors and Downstream Testing: The EISNER (Early Identification of Subclinical Atherosclerosis by Noninvasive Imaging Research) Prospective Randomized Trial. *JACC*, Apr 15;57(15).

Salonen, R. S. (1988). Prevalence of carotid atherosclerosis and serum cholesterol levels in eastern Finland. *Arteriosclerosis*, 8(6), 788-792. doi:10.1161/01. atv.8.6.788.

Scheel, P. M. (2019). Lipoprotein(A) in Clinical Practice. *Am Col Cardio*, July 2.

Shapiro, M. F. (2017). Apolipoprotein B-containing lipoproteins and atherosclerotic cardiovascular disease. *F1000Research*, 6(F1000 Faculty Rev)134:3-8.

Silvestro, A. D. (2006). Falsely high ankle-brachial index predicts major amputation in critical limb ischemia. *Vascular Medicine*, 11(2) 69-74.

Simon, A. M. (2010, February). The Value of Carotid Intima-Media Thickness for Predicting Cardiovascular Risk. *Arterioscler Thromb Vasc Biol.*, 30, 182-185. doi:10.1161/ATVBAHA.109.196980

Sirovich, B. W. (2011). Too Little? Too Much? Primary Care Physicians' Views on US Health Care. *Arch Intern Med*, 171(17): 1582-1585.

Smulders, Y. J. (2000). Cardiovascular autonomic function is associated with (micro)albuminuria in elderly Caucasian subjects with impaired glucose tolerance or type 2 diabetes: The Hoorn Study. *Diabetes Care*, 23:1369-1374.

Sohal, R. W. (1996). Oxidative stress, caloric restriction, and aging. *Science*, 273:59-63.

Stanford Medicine. (2019). Introduction to Measuring the Ankle Brachial Index. *http://stanfordmedicine25.stanford.edu/the25/ankle-brachial-index.html*.

Stehouwer, C. (2004). Endothelial dysfunction in diabetic nephropathy: State of the art and potential significance for non-diabetic renal disease [Editorial]. *Nephrol Dial Transplant*, 19:778-781.

Stehouwer, C. H. (2004). Microalbuminuria is associated with impaired brachial artery, flow-mediated vasodilation in elderly individuals without and with diabetes:Further evidence for a link between microalbuminuria and endothelial dysfunction. The Hoorn Study. *Kidney Int*, 66[Suppl 92]: S42-S44.

Stehouwer, C. S. (2006). Microalbuminuria and risk for CV disease: Analysis of potential mechanisms. *JASN,* 17(8)2106-11.

Stein, J. (2011). Carotid Intima-Media Thickness Progression and Cardiovascular Disease Risk. *JACC*, 57(22): 2011.

Swirski FK, N. M. (2013). Leukocyte behavior in atherosclerosis, myocardial infarction, and heart failure. *Science*, 339(6116): 161-166.

Taylor, A. K. (2002, Oct 15). ARBITER: Arterial Biology for the Investigation of the Treatment Effects of Reducing Cholesterol. *Circulation,* 106(16), 2055-2060.

The SCOT-HEART investigators. (2015). *Lancet*, 385:2283-91.

Tomiyama, H., & Yamashina, A. (2010). Non-Invasive Vascular Function Tests: Their Pathophysiological Background and Clinical Application. *Circulation,* 74: 24-33.

Tsimikas, S. G. (2019). Statin therapy increases lipoprotein levels. *Eur Heart J.*

Tu, J. H. (1998). The Fall & Rise of Carotid Endarterectomy in the US & Canada. *New England Journal of Medicine*, 339:1441-1447.

Turco, J. e. (2018). Cardiovascular Health Promotion An Issue That Can No Longer Wait. . *JACC*, Vol 72(8).

Tuzcu EM, K. S. (2001). High prevalence of coronary atherosclerosis in asymptomatic teenagers and young adults: evidence from intravascular ultrasound. *Circulation*, 103:2705-10.

USPSTF. (2018). Risk Assessment for Cardiovascular Disease With Nontraditional Risk Factors. *JAMA*, 320(3):272-280.

Verma, G. Z. (2008). Surgical difficulties for Total Knee Replacement in Stickler syndrome: A case report. *Cases J.*, 1(1):179.

Virchow, R. (1856). *Phlogose und Thrombose im Gefassystem*. Frankfurt-am-Main: Meidinger Sohn and Company.

Vlachopoulos, C. I. (2015). Biomarkers, erectile dysfunction, and cardiovascular risk prediction: the latest of an evolving concept. *Asian J Androl*, 17(1):17-20.

Weindruch, R. (1997). Caloric Intake and Aging. *NEJM*, 337(14): 986-994.

Wilde, C. (2003). Hidden Causes of Heart Attack and Stroke: Inflammation, Cardiology's New Frontier. *Abingdon Press*, 182-183.

BIBLIOGRAPHY

Willeit, P. T. (2021). Carotid Intima-Media Thickness Progression as Surrogate Marker for Cardiovascular Risk. *Circulation*(142), 621-642. doi:10.1161/CIRCULATIONAHA.120.046361

Yong, P. S. (2010). The Healthcare Imperative. Lowering Costs and Improving Outcomes. IOM Roundtable. *Institute of Medicine of the National Academies.*

Zheng, Z. S. (1997). Associations of ankle-brachial index with clinical coronary heart disease, stroke, and preclinical carotid and popliteal atherosclerosis: the Atherosclerosis Risk in Communities (ARIC) Study. *Atherosclerosis,* (131):115-125.

CPSIA information can be obtained
at www.ICGtesting.com
Printed in the USA
LVHW081916220721
693426LV00003B/36